Federal
HEALTH INFORMATION
Resources

Federal
HEALTH
INFORMATION
Resources™

Edited by Melvin S. Day
Compiled by the Staff of Herner and Company

 INFORMATION RESOURCES PRESS
Arlington, Virginia
1987

Available from
Information Resources Press
1700 North Moore Street
Suite 700
Arlington, Virginia 22209

Library of Congress Catalog Card Number 86-83158

ISBN 0-87815-055-2

Preface

The purpose of this first edition of *Federal Health Information Resources* (*FHIR*) is to bring together in a simple, fully indexed, easy-to-use volume the major sources of biomedical and health information produced or maintained by agencies or contractors of the Federal Government. There are hundreds of such information sources, some broadly known and used and others with extremely narrow constituencies and limited use. Thus, the purpose and impetus for *FHIR* are to inform the reader of probable sources of required or potentially useful health-related information within the federal community and, in small measure, to help stimulate and increase the use of these sources. Two oft-overlooked facts regarding federally supported programs are that their significance and justification are directly proportional to their use; their ultimate goal is (or should be) to reach the largest possible clientele with the smallest possible cost per use.

FHIR is primarily an amalgam of four sources: *Health Information Resources in the Federal Government* and its related database, DIRLINE (DIRECTORY OF INFORMATION RESOURCES ONLINE); the records of the National Referral Center of the Library of Congress Science and Technology Division; information source directories maintained by federal departments and agencies; and intelligence garnered directly from specific federal information activities. Many of the source descriptions so obtained are inevitably dated, but we tried to make them as timely and accurate as possible. In addition to the sympathy and forbearance of our readers, we ask that they call to our attention any inaccuracies or omissions they uncover so that we may remedy them in the second edition of *FHIR*, which we are planning to publish in 1989. We would also appreciate the names of any health-related federal information resources that we may have omitted.

In the course of checking the completeness and accuracy of entries, we found that some information sources ceased to exist or had changed significantly in their locations, affiliations, services, products, or other respects. We attempted to update those entries or, where cessations occurred, tried to identify and direct the reader to a successor source. Again, we solicit the assistance of our readers in calling our attention to changes in the source descriptions.

While the compilers and editor of this first edition of *FHIR* are responsible for its contents, good and bad, we want to acknowledge the contribution of the various informants, institutional and individual, who helped us construct it. These include the compilers of *Health Information Resources in the Federal Government;* the staff of the Science and Technology Division of the Library of Congress, and most particularly its Director, Joseph W. Price, and Staffan Rosenborg, formerly Head of the Publication Section, National Referral Center; and the staffs of the various federal information sources who provided guidance and timely advice regarding their activities.

Finally, we owe a special debt of gratitude to Gene P. Allen, who oversaw the steps involved in taking *FHIR* from a rough (and frequently incorrect, inconsistent, or incomplete) manuscript to its present finished stage, and did so under severe time constraints. We are also appreciative of the efforts of Julie Plumstead Phillips, who prepared the Subject/Title Index; Moo Im Kang, who had to master the intricacies of a new in-house electronic composing system very rapidly, in order to format page layout and get the book composed in time to meet our publication schedule; and Louise Groves and Alice Austin for keyboarding it into computer-readable form.

Contents

Acronyms

The acronyms listed are those used in *FHIR*. Small capital letters denote databases.

ACYF	Administration for Children, Youth, and Families
ADAMHA	Alcohol, Drug Abuse, and Mental Health Administration
ADD	Administration on Developmental Disabilities
AFIP	Armed Forces Institute of Pathology
AFRRI	Armed Forces Radiobiology Research Institute
AFWAL	Air Force Wright Aeronautical Laboratories
AGRICOLA	AGRICULTURE ON-LINE ACCESS
AIDS	Acquired Immune Deficiency Syndrome
AOAC	Association of Official Analytical Chemists
AVLINE	AUDIOVISUALS ONLINE
AVRS	Audiovisual Resources Section
BHCDA	Bureau of Health Care Delivery and Assistance
CAMI	Civil Aeromedical Institute
CANCERLIT	CANCER LITERATURE
CANCERPROJ	CANCER RESEARCH PROJECTS
CAS	Chemical Abstracts Service
CASP	Center for Advanced Study in Pathology
CATLINE	CATALOG ONLINE
CCRIS	CHEMICAL CARCINOGENESIS RESEARCH INFORMATION SYSTEM

CDC	Centers for Disease Control
CEIC	Chemical Effects Information Center
CHAMPUS	Civilian Health and Medical Program of the Uniformed Services
CHEMLINE	CHEMICAL DICTIONARY ONLINE
CHID	COMBINED HEALTH INFORMATION DATABASE
CHPE	Center for Health Promotion and Education
CIC	Consumer Information Center
CIS	Cancer Information Service
CLINPROT	CLINICAL CANCER PROTOCOLS
CPSC	Consumer Product Safety Commission
DARPIS	Drug Abuse Research Project Information System
(D)ED	Department of Education
DHHS	Department of Health and Human Services
DIRLINE	DIRECTORY OF INFORMATION RESOURCES ONLINE
DNA	Deoxyribonucleic Acid
DOD	Department of Defense
DOE	Department of Energy
DRACON	Drug Abuse Communications Network
DRG	Diagnosis-Related Group
EPA	Environmental Protection Agency
ETIC	Environmental Teratology Information Center
FAA	Federal Aviation Administration
FBI	Federal Bureau of Investigation
FDA	Food and Drug Administration
FIC	Federal Information Center
FOI	Freedom of Information Act
FSIS	Food Safety and Inspection Service
FTC	Federal Trade Commission
GAO	General Accounting Office
GPO	U.S. Government Printing Office
HBPIC	High Blood Pressure Information Center
HCFA	Health Care Financing Administration
HHS	Health and Human Services
HISTLINE	HISTORY OF MEDICINE ONLINE
HMO	Health Maintenance Organization
HNIS	Human Nutrition Information Service
HNRIM	HUMAN NUTRITION RESEARCH AND INFORMATION MANAGEMENT
HRSA	Health Resources and Services Administration
HSDB	HAZARDOUS SUBSTANCES DATA BANK
HUD	Department of Housing and Urban Development
ICIC	International Cancer Information Center

ICRP	International Commission on Radiological Protection
IHS	Indian Health Service
ILO	International Labor Organization
IRCC	Information Response to Chemical Concerns
IUD	Intrauterine Device
LAIR	Letterman Army Institute of Research
LC	Library of Congress
LEWS	Loan Early Warning System
MAMC	Madigan Army Medical Center
MECAP	Medical Examiners and Coroners Alert Program
MEDLARS	MEDICAL LITERATURE ANALYSIS AND RETRIEVAL SYSTEM
MEDLINE	MEDLARS ONLINE
MINET	MEDICAL INFORMATION NETWORK
MTF	Medical Treatment Facility
NAL	National Agricultural Library
NAMSIC	National Arthritis and Musculoskeletal and Skin Diseases Information Clearinghouse
NARIC	National Rehabilitation Information Center
NCALI	National Clearinghouse for Alcohol Information
NCEMCH	National Center for Education in Maternal and Child Health
NCHS	National Center for Health Statistics
NCI	National Cancer Institute
NCPCI	National Clearinghouse for Primary Care Information
NCRPM	National Council on Radiation Protection and Measurement
NCTR	National Center for Toxicological Research
NDDIC	National Digestive Diseases Information Clearinghouse
NDIC	National Diabetes Information Clearinghouse
NDN	National Diffusion Network
NEI	National Eye Institute
NEISS	National Electronic Injury Surveillance System
NHPIC	National Health Planning Information Center
NHRC	Naval Health Research Center
NHSC	National Health Service Corps
NHTSA	National Highway Traffic Safety Administration
NIAID	National Institute of Allergy and Infectious Diseases
NICODARD	National Information Center on Orphan Drugs and Rare Diseases
NIDA	National Institute on Drug Abuse
NIDDK	National Institute of Diabetes and Digestive and Kidney Diseases
NIDR	National Institute of Dental Research

NIEHS	National Institute of Environmental Health Sciences
NIH	National Institutes of Health
NIMH	National Institute of Mental Health
NINCDS	National Institute of Neurological and Communicative Disorders and Stroke
NIOSH	National Institute for Occupational Safety and Health
NLM	National Library of Medicine
NLS	National Library Service
NMRI	Naval Medical Research Institute
NTIS	National Technical Information Service
OCA	Office of Consumer Affairs
OCC	Office of Cancer Communications
ODPHP	Office of Disease Prevention and Health Promotion
OEGEP	Office of Economic Growth and Employment Projections
OHDS	Office of Human Development Services
OHF	Office of Health Facilities
OHRR	Office of Health Research Reports
OIH	Office of International Health
OPM	Office of Personnel Management
ORNL	Oak Ridge National Laboratory
OSHA	Occupational Safety and Health Administration
OTA	Office of Technology Assessment
PCMR	President's Committee on Mental Retardation
PCPFS	President's Council on Physical Fitness and Sports
PDQ	PHYSICIAN DATA QUERY
PHE	Patient Health Education
PHS	Public Health Service
POPLINE	POPULATION INFORMATION ONLINE
R&D	Research and Development
RD&E	Research, Development, and Engineering
RAUS	Research Analysis and Utilization System
RML	Regional Medical Library
RSA	Rehabilitation Services Administration
RTECS	REGISTRY OF TOXIC EFFECTS OF CHEMICAL SUBSTANCES
SDILINE	SELECTIVE DISSEMINATION OF INFORMATION ONLINE
SERLINE	SERIALS ONLINE
SIDS	Sudden Infant Death Syndrome
SRP	Scientific Review Panel
TDB	TOXICOLOGY DATA BANK
TIC	Technical Information Center
TIP	Toxicology Information Program
TIRC	Toxicology Information Response Center

TOXLINE	TOXICOLOGY INFORMATION ONLINE
TOXNET	TOXICOLOGY DATA NETWORK
UCLA	University of California, Los Angeles
USDA	Department of Agriculture
VA	Veterans Administration
VALNET	Veterans Administration Library Network

Notes on the Structure and Contents of FHIR

INFORMATION RESOURCES

The source descriptions comprising this section of *FHIR* are catego-
rized by broad subjects (Aerospace Medicine, Cancer Research and
Treatment) and then by official resource names (AFWAL Technical
Library, Argonne National Laboratory), which appear in boldfaced
capital letters. In addition to the source name, each description
contains the parent or generic agency name(s), address, telephone
number, and (where pertinent) subject scope, services, holdings,
databases, and publications.

APPENDIX – DATABASES DESCRIBED IN *FHIR*

The descriptions of the databases that appear in the APPENDIX
are exact duplicates of those that appear in the INFORMATION
RESOURCES section of *FHIR*. Thus, readers who are interested
only in databases will obtain full information from the APPENDIX.
The entry number for each parent resource is, however, included
within each description to provide context and further information,
where required.

INDEXES

The prefix 87- is omitted from the entry numbers in the indexes, since the only purpose of this prefix is to date each entry in the database from which the printed *FHIR* is produced and to aid in the preparation of future editions.

AGENCY / ORGANIZATION INDEX

This index includes entries for agencies or organizational entities that are *official resource names* (primary entries) and those that are *mentioned* within source descriptions or included in their addresses (secondary entries). The primary entries appear in capital letters, and their entry numbers appear immediately following, in italics. The secondary entries that are mentioned only within the source descriptions appear in upper- and lowercase type, and their entry numbers are not italicized. To save space and to make this index as uncluttered as possible, the most numerous parent or generic agency names (Department of Health and Human Services, Public Health Service, National Institutes of Health) are deleted unless these agencies *directly* operate information resources.

SUBJECT / TITLE INDEX

The entries in this index, which include subject terms and titles of publications (italicized), are alphabetized letter-by-letter. The index is thoroughly cross-referenced to foster access to resource descriptions from every user viewpoint. Access is also facilitated through indexing by all subjects covered by each source.

Information Resources

AEROSPACE MEDICINE

87-001 AEROSPACE MEDICAL DIVISION HEADQUARTERS
STINFO Office (RDO)
Department of the Air Force
Air Force Systems Command
Brooks Air Force Base, TX 78235-5000
(512) 536-2838

SERVICES: The division's areas of interest include aerospace medicine, environmental toxicology, radiation hazards, mechanical forces, man-machine integration technology, advanced crew technology, training design and delivery, and aircrew training. The division answers inquiries concerning the status and location of current research projects at Aerospace Medical Division laboratories; specific technical inquiries and requests for reports are referred to the appropriate laboratory. The Museum of Flight Medicine, located at Division Headquarters, is a central depository for memorabilia relating to aerospace medicine from its earliest beginnings to the present.
PUBLICATIONS: Technical reports, technical papers, special reports, and bibliographies.

87-002 AFWAL TECHNICAL LIBRARY
Department of the Air Force
Air Force Systems Command
Air Force Wright Aeronautical Laboratories
AFWAL/GLISL
Wright-Patterson Air Force Base, OH 45433
(513) 255-3630

SERVICES: The library makes interlibrary loans (except reports that are available from the Defense Technical Information Center and the National Technical Information Service). It permits on-site reference service by government contractors, industry representatives, and students.

HOLDINGS: The library's comprehensive collection of more than 118,000 books and bound periodicals, 1,300 journal subscriptions, and thousands of governmental and intergovernmental reports concentrates on all aspects of the aeronautical and aerospace sciences, including aerospace medicine.

87-003 **ARMY AEROMEDICAL RESEARCH LABORATORY**
Department of the Army
Office of the Surgeon General
Army Medical Research and Development Command
P.O. Box 577
Fort Rucker, AL 36362-5292
(205) 255-6907 and 255-6936

SERVICES: Areas of interest include aviation medicine, physiology, orthopedics, physiological optics, biomechanics, biophysics, biochemistry, and psychology; medical aspects of selection, retention, and training of airmen; environment of current and prototype aircraft, including toxicological hazards, thermal stress, sound pressure levels, and other physiological stressors; and health hazard assessments of soldiers' occupational environments and life support equipment. The laboratory answers inquiries; provides consulting, reference, and literature-searching services; and makes interlibrary loans.

87-004 **CIVIL AEROMEDICAL INSTITUTE (CAMI)**
Department of Transportation
Federal Aviation Administration
AAM-100
P.O. Box 25082
Oklahoma City, OK 73125
(405) 686-4806

SERVICES: The institute's principal areas of interest are aviation medicine, including aviation psychology, bioengineering, accident investigation, aeromedical education, occupational health, industrial hygiene engineering, and medical aspects of civil aviation safety; biostatistics in human factors evaluations; impact and acceleration stress; medical certification; general and forensic toxicology; pharmacology; biochemistry; pathology; and radiobiology. It answers inquiries, provides consulting services, and makes referrals to other sources of information. Services are provided free and are available to anyone with a legitimate interest or need-to-know.

DATABASES: CAMI maintains two computerized in-house databases: The Airline Cabin Safety Data Bank contains data on in-flight and emergency evacuation injuries of passengers and crew members. The Air Traffic Control Specialist Database contains data of medical interest to the institute on air traffic control specialist selection, training, and tracking. Inquiries should be addressed to the institute.

87-005 NAVAL AEROSPACE MEDICAL INSTITUTE
Library
Department of the Navy
Naval Medical Command
Bldg. 1953
Pensacola, FL 32508-5600
(904) 452-2256

SERVICES: The mission of the Naval Aerospace Medical Institute is to provide professional technical support and consultative services in operationally related fleet and fleet marine force medical matters worldwide, as well as educational and training programs for medical department personnel in operational medical disciplines. Its areas of interest include aerospace medicine, aviation medicine, military medicine, motion sickness, altitude, adaptation (physiology), naval training, and performance (human). The institute's library provides answers to queries, referral services, and interlibrary loans, primarily to the medical profession, including medical students.

PUBLICATIONS: Institute reports are available from the National Technical Information Service, Springfield, VA 22161.

87-006   **NAVAL AEROSPACE MEDICAL RESEARCH**
         LABORATORY
         Department of the Navy
         Naval Medical Research and Development Command
         Naval Air Station
         Pensacola, FL 32508-5700
         (904) 452-3286

SERVICES: The Naval Aerospace Medical Research Laboratory conducts research and development in aerospace medicine and related scientific areas applicable to aerospace systems. The laboratory's areas of interest are aerospace medicine, aviation medicine, military medicine, motion sickness, vestibular apparatus, altitude, electromagnetic radiation, adaptation (physiology), motor reactions, and radiation hazards. It answers queries, provides referral services, and makes interlibrary loans.

PUBLICATIONS: Laboratory reports are available from the National Technical Information Service, Springfield, VA 22161.

AGING

87-007 **ADMINISTRATION ON AGING**
DIVISION OF TECHNICAL INFORMATION AND
  DISSEMINATION
Department of Health and Human Services
Office of the Assistant Secretary for Human Development
  Services
330 Independence Ave., SW, Rm. 4746
Washington, DC 20201
(202) 245-0641

SERVICES: The division answers telephone and written inquiries dealing with the social and economic well-being of elderly Americans, including benefits, living arrangements, demographic data, "Meals on Wheels" program management, and gerontological health.
PUBLICATION: *Aging Magazine* (bimonthly).

87-008 **GERONTOLOGY RESEARCH CENTER**
Department of Health and Human Services
National Institutes of Health
National Institute on Aging
4940 Eastern Ave.
Baltimore, MD 21224
(301) 955-1707 (Information Office)
(301) 955-1729 (Library)

SERVICES: The center's research interests include biomedical, behavioral, and social research on the aging process and the diseases and other special problems and needs of the aged, including the biology of aging, cognitive changes with age, societal implications of an increase in the average life expectancy, and immunologic competence in aging. The Information Office answers inquiries, distributes publications, and makes referrals to other sources of information. Its services are free and available to the public. The Gerontology Research Center's library answers inquiries; provides reference, literature-searching, and referral services; and makes interlibrary loans. Most of its services are provided free to government officials. Research investigators from other institutions and students are permitted to use its collections on-site during business hours, but photocopying is not available. Tours of the Gerontology Research Center can be arranged with advance notice.

PUBLICATIONS: Books, pamphlets, reports, and studies. A publications list is available on request.

87-009   HUD USER
P.O. Box 280
Germantown, MD 20874-0280
(301) 251-5154

SERVICES: HUD USER, a service of the Office of Policy Development and Research, Department of Housing and Urban Development (HUD), is an in-house computerized information service designed to disseminate the results of research sponsored by HUD. Services include personalized literature searches of the computerized database, document delivery, and special products such as topical bibliographies and announcements of important future research. Health-related topics covered in the HUD USER database include housing safety, housing for the elderly and handicapped, and lead-based paint. There is a handling fee for all documents ordered from HUD USER; please call for charges before ordering.

PUBLICATION: *Recent Research Results* (monthly bulletin).

87-010   NATIONAL INSTITUTE ON AGING
Public Affairs Office

Department of Health and Human Services
National Institutes of Health
Bldg. 31, Rm. 5C-35
9000 Rockville Pike
Bethesda, MD 20892
(301) 496-1752
(301) 495-3455 (Publications Distribution)

SERVICES: The National Institute on Aging was established in 1974 to conduct and support biomedical, social, and behavioral research and training related to the aging process and the diseases and other special problems and needs of the aged. The institute provides for the study of biomedical, psychological, social, educational, and economic aspects of aging through in-house research conducted at its Gerontology Research Center (87-008) in Baltimore, Maryland and through grant support of extramural and collaborative research programs at universities, hospitals, medical centers, and nonprofit institutions throughout the nation. The institute also provides support to institutions that train scientists for research careers in aging.

PUBLICATIONS: Consumer materials are available on menopause, nutrition, arthritis, cancer, aging, Alzheimer's disease, constipation, crime, diabetes, exercise, hearing, high blood pressure, osteoporosis, medicines, senility, flu, urinary incontinence, Chinese-language materials, skin care, and dental care. Professional materials are available on Alzheimer's disease and self-help groups. A publications list is available on request.

ALCOHOL ABUSE, DRUG ABUSE, AND
MENTAL HEALTH

87-011 NATIONAL CLEARINGHOUSE FOR ALCOHOL
INFORMATION (NCALI)
P.O. Box 2345
Rockville, MD 20852
(301) 468-2600

SERVICES: The clearinghouse, established in 1972, gathers and disseminates current knowledge on alcohol-related subjects. Services include subject searches of an in-house automated database, packaged bibliographies on frequently requested subjects, and referrals to treatment and counseling organizations. Books, newsletters, journals, and studies are available for public use in the library, which is located at 1776 East Jefferson Street, Rockville, Maryland. NCALI is a service of the National Institute on Alcohol Abuse and Alcoholism.

DATABASE: The in-house computerized bibliographic Alcohol Information Database, established in 1972, includes abstracts of 50,000 items. Sources indexed by this database include scholarly journals, books, and statistical data. Access to the database is through NCALI.

PUBLICATIONS: Consumer materials are available on fetal alcohol syndrome, alcohol use, alcohol abuse, the elderly, Native Americans, black Americans, and Hispanics. Professional materials are available on fetal alcohol syndrome, alcohol use, and alcohol abuse. A publications list is available.

87-012 ALCOHOL, DRUG ABUSE, AND MENTAL HEALTH
ADMINISTRATION (ADAMHA)

OFFICE OF COMMUNICATIONS AND PUBLIC AFFAIRS
Department of Health and Human Services
Parklawn Bldg., Rm. 12C-15
5600 Fishers Lane
Rockville, MD 20857
(301) 443-3783

SERVICES: Inquiries on alcohol, drug abuse, and mental health can be directed to this office. Requests for publication lists and specific titles should be made directly to the National Clearinghouse for Alcohol Information (87-011), the National Clearinghouse for Drug Abuse Information (87-068), or the National Institute of Mental Health, Public Inquiries Section (87-138).

PUBLICATION: *ADAMHA News* (monthly).

ARTHRITIS, DIABETES, DIGESTIVE, AND KIDNEY DISEASES

87-013 NATIONAL ARTHRITIS AND MUSCULOSKELETAL AND SKIN DISEASES INFORMATION CLEARINGHOUSE (NAMSIC)
P.O. Box 9782
Arlington, VA 22209
(703) 558-4999

SERVICES: The clearinghouse is designed to help health professionals identify print and audiovisual educational materials concerning arthritis and musculoskeletal and skin diseases and to serve as an information exchange for individuals and organizations involved in public, professional, and patient education. Requests are answered by searching the clearinghouse's database and other bibliographic sources and by making referrals to appropriate resources. The clearinghouse is a service of the National Institute of Arthritis and Musculoskeletal and Skin Diseases, DHHS (87-016).

DATABASE: The ARTHRITIS INFORMATION database, begun in 1979, now includes records for more than 5,000 documents published since 1975; approximately 1,000 records are added each year. A thesaurus is used to index the entries. The file is part of the COMBINED HEALTH INFORMATION DATABASE (CHID), accessible to the public through BRS.

PUBLICATIONS: Materials are available on arthritis, musculoskeletal diseases, skin diseases, rheumatic diseases (rheumatoid arthritis, osteoarthritis, systemic lupus erythematosus, scleroderma, Lyme disease, gout, and ankylosing spondylitis), biofeedback, nutrition, pharmaceuticals, patient education, and psychosocial and sexual aspects. NAMSIC *Memo* (irregular announcement). A publications list is available.

87-014 NATIONAL DIABETES INFORMATION CLEARINGHOUSE (NDIC)
P.O. Box NDIC
Bethesda, MD 20205
(301) 468-2162

SERVICES: Established in 1978, NDIC, a service of the National Institute of Diabetes and Digestive and Kidney Diseases (NIDDK), DHHS, collects and disseminates information about patient education materials and programs and is a facilitator in the development of materials for diabetes education. The clearinghouse maintains a meeting registry that includes regional, national, and international meetings, congresses, and symposia of interest to the diabetes community. NDIC distributes its own publications, as well as other diabetes-related materials. A library collection of approximately 4,000 items is open to the public; however, materials do not circulate.

DATABASE: NDIC maintains the online DIABETES INFORMATION database of patient education and professional materials. It is a component of the COMBINED HEALTH INFORMATION DATABASE (CHID), accessible to the public through BRS. Indexing is based on a thesaurus developed by the clearinghouse.

PUBLICATIONS: Consumer materials are available on diabetes, foot care, nutrition, insulin, blood glucose monitoring, elderly Americans, and eye care. Professional materials are available on diabetes, pregnancy, patient education, exercise, nutrition, diabetic retinopathy, and foot care.

87-015 NATIONAL DIGESTIVE DISEASES INFORMATION CLEARINGHOUSE (NDDIC)
1255 23rd St., NW, Suite 275
Washington, DC 20037
(202) 296-1138

SERVICES: The clearinghouse, a service of the National Institute of Diabetes and Digestive and Kidney Diseases (NIDDK), DHHS, was established in 1980 as the National Digestive Diseases Education and Information Clearinghouse to provide a central information and education resource on digestive health and the prevention and management of digestive diseases. It develops, identifies, and distributes educational materials; encourages production of needed materials; and responds to requests for information.

DATABASE: The DIGESTIVE DISEASES PATIENT EDUCATION MATERIALS database contains information about the clearinghouse's patient education materials and is a part of the COMBINED HEALTH INFORMATION DATABASE (CHID), which is accessible to the public through BRS.

PUBLICATIONS: Consumer materials are available on cirrhosis, diarrhea, gallstone disease, dyspepsia, digestive diseases, heartburn, hiatal hernia, hydrogen breath test, hepatitis B, ulcers, ulcerative colitis, irritable bowel syndrome, and Crohn's disease. Professional materials are available on digestive diseases, gallstones, chenodiol, biliary cirrhosis, Crohn's disease, endoscopy, neonatal hepatitis, and liver transplantation.

**87-016   NATIONAL INSTITUTE OF ARTHRITIS AND
          MUSCULOSKELETAL AND SKIN DISEASES
          INFORMATION OFFICE**
Department of Health and Human Services
National Institutes of Health
Bldg. 31, Rm. 9A-04
9000 Rockville Pike
Bethesda, MD 20892
(301) 496-3583

SERVICES: Inquiries relating to the following conditions and diseases for which the institute is responsible are handled by its Information Office: arthritis, bone diseases, and skin diseases. Requests for certain publications are handled by the National Arthritis and Musculoskeletal and Skin Diseases Information Clearinghouse (87-013).

PUBLICATIONS: Consumer materials are available on arthritis, epidermolysis bullosa, osteoporosis, and vitiligo. Professional materials are available on arthritis and systemic lupus erythematosus.

**87-017   NATIONAL INSTITUTE OF DIABETES AND DIGESTIVE
AND KIDNEY DISEASES (NIDDK)
OFFICE OF HEALTH RESEARCH REPORTS**
Department of Health and Human Services
National Institutes of Health
Bldg. 31, Rm. 9A-04
9000 Rockville Pike
Bethesda, MD 20892
(301) 496-3583

SERVICES: The Office of Health Research Reports (OHRR) has oversight management responsibility for two information clearinghouses and for a new one to be established. The two ongoing clearinghouses are: the National Diabetes Information Clearinghouse (87-014) and the National Digestive Diseases Information Clearinghouse (87-015). The new clearinghouse will be called the National Kidney and Urologic Diseases Information Clearinghouse. OHRR manages a major publications program.

PUBLICATIONS: Publications on diabetes, digestive, and kidney diseases and related health matters. Inquiries from professionally qualified persons regarding health-related publications, data, and information should be directed to OHRR.

BASIC BIOMEDICAL SCIENCES RESEARCH

87-018 BROOKHAVEN NATIONAL LABORATORY
Research Library
Upton, NY 11973
(516) 282-3490

SERVICES: The Brookhaven National Laboratory, operated
for the Department of Energy, conducts basic research in (1)
medical sciences, including industrial medicine, microbiology,
biochemistry, physiology, medical physics, and hematology; (2)
physics, including high energy physics, structural and theoret-
ical physics, neutron physics and nuclear structure, solid state
physics, and low-energy physics; (3) chemistry, including nuclear chemistry, inorganic chemistry, radiation and hot atom
chemistry, isotope effects, analytical chemistry, and physical
chemistry; (4) biology, including genetics, general physiology,
biochemistry, biophysics, molecular biology, and ecology; and
(5) instrumentation and health physics. Collections of the library include 90,000 books, 2,000 current periodicals, 500,000
reports, and 60,000 volumes of bound journals. The Research
Library accesses a wide variety of U.S. government and commercial computerized databases. Using this comprehensive information resource, the library answers brief inquiries, provides
limited reference services, makes interlibrary loans, and permits
on-site use of its collection by appointment.

**87-019 NATIONAL INSTITUTE OF GENERAL MEDICAL
          SCIENCES
          OFFICE OF RESEARCH REPORTS**
Department of Health and Human Services

National Institutes of Health
Bldg. 31, Rm. 4A-52
9000 Rockville Pike
Bethesda, MD 20892
(301) 496-7301

SERVICES: The Office of Research Reports responds to inquiries relating to the institute's research activities in the basic biomedical sciences. The institute's program areas include cellular and molecular bases of disease, genetics, pharmacological sciences, biophysics and physiological sciences, and minority access to research careers. Information on types of research and research training support available for institutions and individuals may be obtained from the Office of Research Reports, which also disseminates publications.

PUBLICATIONS: Consumer materials are available on medicines, basic research, and cell biology. Professional materials are available on research grants and training programs, basic research, burn and trauma research, genetics, and genetic diseases.

BIOMEDICAL COMMUNICATIONS RESEARCH

87-020 **LISTER HILL NATIONAL CENTER FOR BIOMEDICAL COMMUNICATIONS**
Department of Health and Human Services
National Institutes of Health
National Library of Medicine
Bldg. 38A, Rm. 7N-707
8600 Rockville Pike
Bethesda, MD 20894
(301) 496-4441

SERVICES: The Lister Hill National Center for Biomedical Communications (including elements of the former National Medical Audiovisual Center) is responsible for conducting research and development in computer-assisted instruction, distributed information systems, artificial intelligence and expert systems, and electronic document storage and retrieval. The center's programs are in six areas: communications engineering, information technology, computer science, audiovisual program development, health professions applications, and training and consultation.

PUBLICATIONS: Reports issued by the center are available from the National Technical Information Service, Springfield, VA 22161. A publications list may be requested from the National Library of Medicine's Office of Inquiries and Publications Management, 8600 Rockville Pike, Bethesda, MD 20894, (301) 496-6308.

BLIND, HANDICAPPED, DISABLED, AND REHABILITATION

87-021 ADMINISTRATION ON DEVELOPMENTAL DISABILITIES (ADD)
Department of Health and Human Services
Office of the Assistant Secretary for Human Development Services
Hubert H. Humphrey Bldg., Rm. 351D
200 Independence Ave., SW
Washington, DC 20201
(202) 245-2890

SERVICES: ADD is responsible for administering the Developmental Disabilities Act, which mandates four grant programs aimed at improving the quality of life for people with developmental disabilities. ADD and State Developmental Disabilities Councils work with other federal, state, and private agencies in serving the needs of physically and mentally disabled citizens. ADD disseminates information through the media, reports, correspondence, and answers to inquiries. It makes basic formula grants to states for planning, coordinating, and administering services, and protection and advocacy formula grants for supporting state systems to protect and advocate for the rights of persons with developmental disabilities. It also makes grants to 36 university-affiliated facilities and 5 satellite centers to support interdisciplinary training of professionals serving developmentally disabled individuals, evaluative and diagnostic services, and research and demonstration projects. Special projects grants are awarded for projects of regional or national significance through a coordinated discretionary grants process. These projects often demonstrate and disseminate information on improved methods of service delivery.

87-022   CLEARINGHOUSE ON THE HANDICAPPED
Department of Education
Office of the Assistant Secretary for Special Education
   and Rehabilitative Services
Mary E. Switzer Bldg., Rm. 3132
330 C St., SW
Washington, DC 20202
(202) 732-1245

SERVICES: The clearinghouse, established in 1975, serves
two purposes: (1) to respond to inquiries from handicapped individuals, and (2) to serve as a resource to organizations that
supply information to and about handicapped persons. Requests
are handled by referring individuals to relevant sources, using
a directory of 300 national information providers and the clearinghouse's files of state and local resources. The library is open
to the public.
PUBLICATIONS: Materials are available on federal funding,
regulations, legislation, and organizations. *Programs for the
Handicapped* (bimonthly newsletter).

**87-023   NATIONAL LIBRARY SERVICE (NLS) FOR THE BLIND
            AND PHYSICALLY HANDICAPPED**
Library of Congress
1291 Taylor St., NW
Washington, DC 20542
(202) 287-5100
(800) 424-8567

SERVICES: Established by Congress in 1931, NLS comprises
a network of 56 regional and 103 local libraries that work in cooperation with the Library of Congress to provide a free library
service to persons who are unable to read or use standard printed
materials because of temporary or permanent visual or physical
impairment.   NLS delivers books and magazines in recorded
form or in braille to eligible readers by postage-free mail and
provides for them to be returned in the same manner. Specially

designed phonographs and cassette players are loaned free to persons borrowing talking books. NLS also provides information on blindness and physical handicaps on request. Persons interested in these services should contact the library serving their area. A list of local and regional libraries is available on request.

PUBLICATIONS: A *Bibliography of Braille* and recorded materials on health topics will be sent on request. *Braille Book Review* (bimonthly); *Talking Book Topics* (bimonthly); and *Update* (quarterly).

87-024 NATIONAL REHABILITATION INFORMATION CENTER (NARIC)
The Catholic University of America
4407 8th St., NE
Washington, DC 20017
(202) 635-5822
(800) 34-NARIC

SERVICES: Established in 1977, NARIC, a service of the National Institute of Disability and Rehabilitation Research (formerly the National Institute of Handicapped Research), Department of Education, supplies publications and audiovisual materials on rehabilitation, prepares bibliographies tailored to specific requests, and assists in locating answers to questions. NARIC's collection includes materials relevant to the rehabilitation of all disability groups, as well as documents relevant to professional and administrative practices and concerns. The collection contains 300 periodical titles and more than 11,000 research reports, books, and audiovisual materials. The public can use the NARIC collection or order materials from the center.

DATABASES: REHABDATA, an online database, includes bibliographic information and abstracts of the entire NARIC collection of 300 periodical titles and more than 11,000 research reports, books, and audiovisuals, including materials produced from 1950 to the present. NARIC also maintains ABLEDATA, an online database of information about more than 4,000 commercially available rehabilitation products useful to persons with disabilities; it also includes a network of brokers. Manufacturers of products for the disabled and those seeking product information are encouraged to use this system. Direct access to both databases is through BRS. The ABLEDATA thesaurus, REHABDATA thesaurus, ABLEDATA search manual, and ABLEDATA reference guide are useful aids for database searching. There is a charge for photoduplication. Customized literature searches of the NARIC databases are available for nominal fees.

PUBLICATIONS: Materials include a periodical holdings list and a subject catalog. *Rehabilitation Research Review* (irregular series).

87-025   **PRESIDENT'S COMMITTEE ON EMPLOYMENT**
            OF THE HANDICAPPED
Public Affairs Division
Vanguard Bldg., Suite 636
1111 20th St., NW
Washington, DC 20036
(202) 653-5044

SERVICES: The committee, established in 1947, strives to eliminate environmental and attitudinal barriers impeding the opportunities and progress of handicapped persons. Among its major activities is an ongoing public information campaign that includes awards programs, films, exhibits, a speakers bureau, and public service advertising. The committee is involved in National Employ the Handicapped Week (the first full week of October). The 12 standing committees include consumer affairs, labor, mentally handicapped, and youth development.

PUBLICATIONS: Materials are available on employment of disabled people, affirmative action, independent living, the Rehabilitation Act (Section 504), taxes and disability, disabled veterans, and job placement. *Disabled USA* (quarterly information bulletin).

87-026 **REHABILITATION SERVICES ADMINISTRATION (RSA)**
Department of Education
Office of the Assistant Secretary for Special Education
  and Rehabilitative Services
Mary E. Switzer Bldg., Rm. 3024
330 C St., SW
Washington, DC 20202
(202) 732-1282

SERVICES: The Rehabilitation Services Administration was created to administer federally sponsored and supported vocational rehabilitation programs for physically and mentally disabled persons. Its State-Federal Vocational Rehabilitation Program includes evaluation and work adjustment services, special projects for handicapped migratory and seasonal farm workers and employers, demonstrations and training programs to increase the supply of rehabilitation personnel, and grants for construction of rehabilitation facilities. Federal law specifies that these services be vocationally oriented and geared to developing the skills and work habits needed to enable the handicapped to obtain jobs in the competitive market. RSA's technical assistance program provides free short-term consultation services to nonprofit rehabilitation facilities to help improve their operations. Other programs administered by RSA include the placement of trained disabled persons in private industry jobs. RSA is also active in programs to remove architectural barriers to the handicapped and in projects that assist clients in their relations with vocational rehabilitation programs.

PUBLICATIONS: Materials available include program information and a list of state vocational rehabilitation agencies. *American Rehabilitation* (quarterly journal).

CANCER RESEARCH AND TREATMENT

87-027   **ARGONNE NATIONAL LABORATORY**
          9700 S. Cass Ave.
          Argonne, IL 60439
          (312) 972-2000

          SERVICES: The Argonne National Laboratory, operated by
          the University of Chicago for the Department of Energy, con-
          ducts basic scientific research. In addition to research and de-
          velopment related to energy systems, its areas of interest also in-
          clude cancer research, genetics, and cellular biology. The Tech-
          nical Information Services Department (312/972-4224) provides
          broad-scope library and technical information to the laboratory
          staff. The Central Library (312/972-4223) handles all interli-
          brary loans. Visitors may use the libraries during normal work-
          ing hours by writing to the library or telephoning 312/972-4223
          or 971-4224. The Office of Public Affairs (312/972-5575) an-
          swers inquiries; handles public information functions; directs a
          technical exhibit program, a lecture service, and an Argonne
          tour service; and distributes educational literature to student re-
          questers.

87-028   **CANCER INFORMATION CLEARINGHOUSE**
          Department of Health and Human Services
          National Institutes of Health
          National Cancer Institute
          9000 Rockville Pike
          Bethesda, MD 20892

          SERVICES: The clearinghouse, begun in 1975, collected in-
          formation on public and patient cancer education materials and

disseminated it to health professionals and health educators. Documents were abstracted, indexed, and stored in an automated storage and retrieval system. The Cancer Information Clearing-house was discontinued on October 1, 1986. Consumer inquiries and queries from health professionals should now be directed to the Office of Cancer Communications (87-034) or the Cancer Information Service (87-029).

DATABASE: The in-house computerized Cancer Education Materials Database contains abstracts of and index entries to public and patient pre-1986 cancer information materials. Maintenance of the database was discontinued in 1986.

87-029   **CANCER INFORMATION SERVICE (CIS)**
Department of Health and Human Services
National Institutes of Health
National Cancer Institute
9000 Rockville Pike
Bethesda, MD 20892-4200
(301) 427-8656 (Project Officer)
(800) 4-Cancer (U.S.A.)
(800) 638-6070 (Alaska)
(800) 524-1234 (Hawaii; neighbor islands call collect)

Located at: Blair Bldg., Rm. 414
8300 Colesville Rd.
Silver Spring, MD 20910

SERVICES: CIS is a toll-free telephone inquiry system that supplies information about cancer and cancer-related resources to the general public and to cancer patients and their families. Callers are automatically put in touch with the office serving their area. Inquiries are handled by health educators and trained volunteers. Spanish-speaking staff members are available to callers from the following areas (daytime hours only): California (area codes 213, 714, and 805), Florida, Georgia, Illinois, northern New Jersey, New York City, and Texas.

PUBLICATIONS: Distributes publications of the National Cancer Institute.

87-030 DIVISION OF CANCER PREVENTION AND CONTROL
Breast Cancer Program
Department of Health and Human Services
National Institutes of Health
National Cancer Institute
9000 Rockville Pike
Bethesda, MD 20892-4200
(301) 427-8818

Located at: Blair Bldg., Rm. 717
8300 Colesville Rd.
Silver Spring, MD 20910

SERVICES: The division's primary areas of interest are human and animal breast cancer, epidemiology, biology of normal and malignant mammary tissue, research in diagnostic procedures, and therapy (radiation, surgery, chemo-, and steroid). It provides reference services, distributes publications on clinical and experimental mammary cancer, and makes referrals to other sources of information. Services are free, primarily for people working in the field of breast cancer.

PUBLICATIONS: *Breast Cancer Task Force Intercom* (monthly bulletin); *Breast Cancer Task Force Program Book* (annual); and bibliographies.

87-031 DIVISION OF CANCER TREATMENT
Department of Health and Human Services
National Institutes of Health
National Cancer Institute
Bldg. 31, Rm. 3A-52
9000 Rockville Pike
Bethesda, MD 20892
(301) 496-4291

SERVICES: The division plans and conducts the organization of technical information on cancer treatment, including information generated by the Cancer Treatment Program and other collaborative research programs, and acts as the focal point for information on the Cancer Treatment Program. The program encompasses direct research as well as surveillance over the world's literature on cancer therapy. The division's areas of interest are cancer therapy, including chemical and biological compounds with an antitumor effect; surgical and radiation therapies; and basic/preclinical research. A hard copy collection of original articles abstracted for *Cancer Therapy Abstracts* is maintained for reference purposes. The division answers inquiries, provides consulting and literature-searching services, and distributes publications at cost. Nonproprietary data are made available on a limited basis to federal agencies and others involved in cancer therapy research, as well as to interested scientists and physicians.

DATABASES: The Cancer Treatment Program maintains a number of computerized in-house databanks of clinical, biological, and chemical information. One major file, the Biological Materials Database, contains raw and evaluated biological data on approximately 675,000 natural and synthetic materials. Another, the Synthetic Chemical Compound Database, contains structural data on 400,000 synthetic compounds, of which, nomenclature information is available on approximately 265,000. The Cancer Treatment Clinical Trials Database contains information on approximately 5,700 clinical trials worldwide.

PUBLICATIONS: The *Journal of the National Cancer Institute (JNCI)* is published monthly for the entire cancer research community. Since it was founded in 1940, *JNCI* has been one of the main channels for dissemination of the latest research findings on progress against cancer. *JNCI* serves primarily to publish new findings related to cancer problems; however, many studies reported in its pages add to basic scientific knowledge and provide leads to solving problems outside the cancer field. Papers in *JNCI* report on the clinical and experimental aspects of cancer research in the following areas: cancer biochemistry, carcinogenesis, immunology and virology, epidemiology, and cancer control and prevention. Although *JNCI* is an official publication of the National Cancer Institute, more than 90 percent of the papers published are from scientists at other research institutions, hospitals, and universities. Approximately one third of the papers published are from researchers outside the United States. *Cancer Treatment Reports (CTR),* a monthly journal, was founded a quarter of a century ago as *Cancer Chemotherapy Reports* and focused on the rapidly expanding study of drugs in the treatment of malignant diseases. In 1976, its name was changed to *Cancer Treatment Reports* in acknowledgement of the coming of age of chemotherapy as an established form of treatment. Over the past few years, *CTR* has been perhaps the most important single source of new information in the area of developmental therapeutics in neoplastic disease. Its contents have spanned the range from drug discovery and design to clinical trials of complex multimodal treatment schemes. The journal has published a large number of important papers on methodologic issues in drug screening, toxicology, pharmacology, and clinical trials of new therapies. Thoughtful reviews on selected topics and stimulating editorials round out the journal's contents. *NCI Monographs* is a publication for the timely reporting of proceedings of key conferences dealing with cancer and closely related research fields or a related group of papers on specific subjects of importance to cancer research. It replaces the former *National Cancer Institute Monograph Series* and *Cancer Treatment Symposia* and serves as a supplement to *JNCI* and *CTR*. Investigators wishing to publish in *NCI Monographs* should contact the editor of one of these two journals. The journals and monographs are available from the Superintendent of Documents, U.S. Government Printing Office, Washington, DC 20402.

87-032   **FREDERICK CANCER RESEARCH FACILITY**
Fermentation Program
Department of Health and Human Services
National Institutes of Health
National Cancer Institute
P.O. Box B
Frederick, MD 21701
(301) 698-1160

SERVICES: This program's principal areas of interest are cancer, chemotherapy, cancer chemotherapeutic agents, and antibiotics.

DATABASE: The program maintains a computerized in-house Antibiotics, Antitumor, and Antiviral Natural Products database that contains more than 10,500 compounds. Comparison of unknown compounds with entries can be made using physical and descriptive characteristics. Service is available to scientific groups for a fee. Queries should be addressed to the facility in Frederick, Maryland.

87-033   INTERNATIONAL CANCER INFORMATION CENTER
(ICIC)
Department of Health and Human Services
National Institutes of Health
National Cancer Institute
Bldg. 82
9030 Old Georgetown Rd.
Bethesda, MD 20892
(301) 496-9096

SERVICES: The International Cancer Information Center is the focal point for dissemination of technical cancer information. Its goal is to make physicians and scientists aware of the most recent and significant developments in the prevention and treatment of cancer. To this end, ICIC develops and applies state-of-the-art computer and telecommunications technology to collect the results of cancer research and to disseminate this information for the benefit of physicians, cancer researchers, and other health professionals throughout the world. The information is provided through computer databases and publications that are timely and easy to use.

DATABASES: The CANCERLINE System of the National Cancer Institute consists of three separate databases: CANCERLIT, CANCERPROJ, and CLINPROT. CANCERLIT (CANCER LITERATURE) contains approximately 500,000 citations and abstracts of published international literature dealing with all aspects of cancer; it is updated monthly with approximately 5,000 abstracts. Approximately 80 percent of the literature is selected from an international collection of 3,000 biomedical and scientific journals. Nonserial literature (including books, reports, and meeting abstracts) contributes the remaining 20 percent. Informative abstracts averaging 200 words are included for most selected cancer-related documents. The database includes cancer literature from 1963 forward. Literature available for the period 1963 through 1976 is limited to references that had been selected for *Carcinogenesis Abstracts* and *Cancer Therapy Abstracts*. In 1977, the scope of the database was expanded to include all cancer-related literature, except most single case histories. In 1980, new records began including *MeSH* terms for uniform retrieval, and since January 1985, new records have been indexed with chemical names and CAS Registry/EC Numbers. CANCERPROJ (CANCER RESEARCH PROJECTS) contains approximately 5,000 descriptions of current cancer research projects around the world. This file was reactivated in April 1985 and is expected to grow steadily, with quarterly updating, toward an eventual size of approximately 10,000 records. It contains descriptions of federally and privately supported grants and contracts. Twenty percent of the project descriptions are provided by scientists from outside the United States. The project summaries are usually divided into a statement of the research objective, a description of the experimental approach, and a statement of any progress made to date. CLINPROT (CLINICAL CANCER PROTOCOLS) contains summaries of approximately 5,000 clinical trials of new anticancer agents or treatment modalities. Updated monthly, most of the protocols in CLINPROT are provided by the Division of Cancer Treatment (87-031) of the National Cancer Institute, while the remaining protocols are provided by major U.S. cancer centers or sources outside the United States. Protocol summaries include the objective and an outline of the study, patient entry criteria, dosage schedules, dosage forms, and special study parameters. The name and telephone number of the study group chairman are provided. CLINPROT is designed primarily as a reference tool for clinical oncologists.

Another link in the National Cancer Institute's efforts to reduce cancer deaths by one half by the year 2000 is PDQ (PHYSICIAN DATA QUERY), an interactive database sponsored by NCI and maintained by ICIC that provides ready access to information on state-of-the-art and investigational cancer treatments. This online information system is designed to more effectively disseminate information on cancer treatment to the medical community. The PDQ database consists of three interlinked files, organized and internally arranged to facilitate interactive searching and retrieval of information by users. These files cover cancer information and treatment, a directory of physicians and organizations that provide cancer care, and active NCI-supported protocols from the CLINPROT file. To each of these approximately 700 research protocol descriptions, NCI has added a list of the institutions where the protocol is being used to treat patients and the name of an oncologist to contact at each institution for information about the protocol. The database is menu-driven, which makes it a "user-friendly" system for individuals who are inexperienced in using computers for online information searching.

All four NCI databases can be accessed through MEDLARS of the National Library of Medicine (87-055).

PUBLICATIONS: *CANCERGRAMS* are monthly current-awareness bulletins containing abstracts of recently published articles on cancer, selected by screening more than 2,000 biomedical publications. Some 60 different *CANCERGRAMS* series are available, collectively affording virtually complete coverage of the entire field of cancer research. The three major subject areas are cancer diagnosis and therapy, carcinogenesis, and cancer virology and immunology. *CANCERGRAMS* can be purchased from the Superintendent of Documents, U.S. Government Printing Office, Washington, DC 20402.

87-034 OFFICE OF CANCER COMMUNICATIONS (OCC)
Department of Health and Human Services
National Institutes of Health
National Cancer Institute
Bldg. 31, Rm. 10A-18

9000 Rockville Pike
Bethesda, MD 20892
(301) 496-5583

SERVICES: Requests for cancer information posed by patients and the public are answered by the Public Inquiries Section
of OCC through distribution of National Cancer Institute publications and by written responses. Additionally, telephone inquiries are received through the Cancer Information Service's
(CIS) (87-029) national toll-free telephone number (800/4-
Cancer). Referrals are made to other sections of OCC or to
CIS, which also responds to inquiries from health professionals
about public and patient education materials.

PUBLICATIONS: Consumer materials are available on breast
cancer, radiation therapy, cancer, cancer prevention, skin cancer,
diethylstilbestrol exposure, chemotherapy, dysplasia, Hodgkin's
disease, leukemia, melanoma, Wilm's tumor, carcinogens,
smoking, and clinical trials. *What You Need to Know About
Cancer* (pamphlet series).

CHEMICAL EFFECTS

87-035   CHEMICAL EFFECTS INFORMATION CENTER (CEIC)
Oak Ridge National Laboratory
Information Research and Analysis Section
Biology Division
Bldg. 2001
P.O. Box X
Oak Ridge, TN 37831
(615) 576-7568

SERVICES: CEIC, operated for the Department of Energy by the Oak Ridge National Laboratory, provides information support to the scientific community concerning the health and environmental effects of chemical pollutants. Its areas of interest are toxic substances, including production and use; chemical and physical properties; metabolism; physiological and toxicological effects; and environmental and ecological effects. The center prepares state-of-the-art reviews and health and environmental assessment reports; develops specialized databases and catalogs; and coordinates and participates in workshops related to CEIC areas of interest.

PUBLICATIONS: The *Reviews* and *Assessment Reports* prepared by the center are available from the National Technical Information Service, Springfield, VA 22161.

CHILDREN, YOUTH, MOTHERS, AND FAMILIES

87-036   **ADMINISTRATION FOR CHILDREN, YOUTH, AND**
         FAMILIES (ACYF)
         Office of Public Affairs
         Department of Health and Human Services
         Office of the Assistant Secretary for Human
           Development Services
         P.O. Box 1182
         Washington, DC 20013
         (202) 472-7257

         Located at: 400 6th St., SW, Rm. 5030
                       Washington, DC 20201

         SERVICES: The Office of Public Affairs for the Office of
         Human Development Services serves as the central information
         resource for the administration.   Inquiries are answered using
         publications from various ACYF offices on the subjects of child
         abuse, day care, and Head Start.   In-depth questions regarding
         child abuse are referred to the Clearinghouse on Child Abuse
         and Neglect Information (87-038).
         PUBLICATION: *Children Today* (bimonthly journal).

87-037   **CENTER FOR RESEARCH FOR MOTHERS AND**
         CHILDREN
         Department of Health and Human Services
         National Institutes of Health
         National Institute of Child Health and Human Development
         9000 Rockville Pike
         Bethesda, MD 20892
         (301) 496-5133 (Office of Research Reporting)

Located at: Landow Bldg., Rm. 7C-03
7910 Woodmont Ave.
Bethesda, MD 20892

SERVICES: The center's principal areas of interest are research and training concerned with investigations of the reproductive processes in man and animals, including fertility behavior and fertility regulation. Special emphasis is placed on reproductive biology, development of new contraceptive methods, and immediate and long-term effects of contraceptive agents. Also emphasized are the problems related to population growth, including effects on the health and well-being of the populations involved, characteristics of populations and their growth rates, responses to population pressures, and studies of how individuals and economic and political institutions react to population dynamics. The center also answers public and professional queries.

87-038   CLEARINGHOUSE ON CHILD ABUSE AND NEGLECT INFORMATION
P.O. Box 1182
Washington, DC 20013
(301) 251-5157

SERVICES: The clearinghouse, established in 1975, collects, processes, and disseminates information on child abuse and neglect and responds to public inquiries. Online searches of its computerized database are conducted, and topical documents, resource materials, and evaluation reports are produced. The document collection of the clearinghouse is open to the public by appointment. The clearinghouse is operated for the National Center on Child Abuse and Neglect, DHHS.
DATABASE: The CHILD ABUSE AND NEGLECT INFORMATION database, begun in 1977, is updated semiannually and primarily covers materials produced between 1965 and the present. Sources indexed by this database include approximately 8,600 published documents, 3,500 program descriptions, 100 descriptions of research projects, and 550 descriptions of audiovisual

materials, as well as excerpts from current state and territorial child abuse and neglect laws, including the welfare, criminal, and juvenile court codes. The database is accessible to the public through DIALOG. A thesaurus is available for a fee.

PUBLICATIONS: Consumer materials are available on child abuse and neglect, sexual abuse, domestic violence, parenting, volunteers, and adolescents. Professional materials are available on program development, domestic violence, crisis intervention, and research activities. Some publications are available free of charge. A publications catalog is available free on request.

87-039   DIVISION OF MATERNAL AND CHILD HEALTH
Bureau of Health Care Delivery and Assistance
Department of Health and Human Services
Office of the Assistant Secretary for Health
Parklawn Bldg., Rm. 6-05
5600 Fishers Lane
Rockville, MD 20857
(301) 443-2170

SERVICES: The division administers grants to state health agencies for maternal and child health and handicapped children's services and to institutions of higher learning for training of health care personnel. Funding is also provided for special projects of regional and national significance. Inquiries related to programs, funding, and available services are handled by the division.

PUBLICATIONS: Professional and consumer publications produced by the division are distributed by the National Maternal and Child Health Clearinghouse (87-043) and the Sudden Infant Death Syndrome Clearinghouse (87-045).

87-040   FAMILY LIFE INFORMATION EXCHANGE
P.O. Box 10716
Rockville, MD 20850
(301) 770-3662

SERVICES: The Family Life Information Exchange, formerly the National Clearinghouse for Family Planning Information, established in 1976, collects family planning materials, conducts searches of its database, makes referrals to other information centers, distributes several Department of Health and Human Services (DHHS) publications, produces materials, and maintains mailing lists of family planning grantees and clinics supported by the Office of Family Planning. The exchange is operated for the Office of Family Planning of the Office of Population Affairs, Public Health Service, DHHS. It primarily serves federally funded family planning clinics.

DATABASE: The exchange maintains an in-house computerized Family Planning Information Database that contains approximately 5,000 entries. The documents and audiovisuals indexed include patient education materials and descriptions of patient education methods.

PUBLICATIONS: Consumer materials are available on contraception, sterilization, and diethylstilbestrol. Professional materials are available on family planning, adolescents, primary care, and infertility. *Health Education Bulletin* (irregular); *Information Service Bulletin* (irregular); and *Directory of Family Planning Grantees, Delegates, and Clinics* (annual). Publications are free in limited quantities. A publications list is available.

87-041   NATIONAL CENTER FOR EDUCATION IN MATERNAL AND CHILD HEALTH
38th and R Sts., NW
Washington, DC 20057
(202) 625-8400

SERVICES: The center provides information and educational assistance, responds to consumer and professional inquiries, provides needs assessments, reviews and evaluates curriculum materials, and develops educational materials focusing on maternal and child health. A library collection of more than 8,000 sources and 50 serials is maintained, and searches of relevant databases are conducted. The center is operated for the Division of Maternal and Child Health (87-039).

PUBLICATIONS: Materials are available on maternal and child health, human genetics, sickle cell anemia, and genetic engineering. *Directory of Clinical Genetic Service Centers—A National Listing* (irregular); *What's New in the NCEMCH Resource Center.*

87-042 NATIONAL INSTITUTE OF CHILD HEALTH AND HUMAN DEVELOPMENT
Office of Research Reporting
Department of Health and Human Services
National Institutes of Health
Bldg. 31, Rm. 2A-32
9000 Rockville Pike
Bethesda, MD 20892
(301) 496-5133

SERVICES: The institute conducts and supports basic and clinical research in maternal and child health and the population sciences. It will respond to individual inquiries on related topics such as studies on reproductive biology and contraception, fertility and infertility, developmental biology and nutrition, mental retardation, and developmental disabilities.

PUBLICATIONS: Consumer materials are available on anorexia nervosa, Cesarean childbirth, Down's syndrome, oral contraception, precocious puberty, premature birth, pregnancy, smoking and pregnancy, vasectomy, childhood hyperactivity, maternal health, and child health. Professional materials are available on sudden infant death syndrome, developmental disabilities, pregnancy, maternal health, child health, and genetics. A publications list is available.

87-043 NATIONAL MATERNAL AND CHILD HEALTH CLEARINGHOUSE
38th and R Sts., NW
Washington, DC 20057
(202) 625-8410

SERVICES: The National Maternal and Child Health Clearinghouse is the centralized source of materials and information in the areas of human genetics and maternal and child health. The clearinghouse responds to inquiries; disseminates approximately 500 titles; and produces fact sheets, topical bibliographies, and referral lists in the field. It is a service of the Division of Maternal and Child Health (87-039).

PUBLICATIONS: Materials are available on breastfeeding, developmental disabilities, phenylketonuria, metabolic disorders, nutrition, prenatal care, and genetic diseases.

87-044   OFFICE OF ADOLESCENT PREGNANCY PROGRAMS
Department of Health and Human Services
Office of the Assistant Secretary for Health
Hubert H. Humphrey Bldg., Rm. 736E
200 Independence Ave., SW
Washington, DC 20201
(202) 245-0142

SERVICES: The primary mission of the Office of Adolescent Pregnancy Programs is to have an impact on the quality of comprehensive care for pregnant adolescents. The office funds demonstration grants to public and private nonprofit organizations and agencies that support positive, family-centered approaches to the problems of adolescent premarital sexual relations, including adolescent pregnancy. The office also funds innovative approaches to the delivery of care services for pregnant adolescents. Primary emphasis is placed on unmarried adolescents who are under 18 years old. The office promotes adoption as an alternative for adolescent parents.

87-045   SUDDEN INFANT DEATH SYNDROME CLEARINGHOUSE
8201 Greensboro Dr., Suite 600
McLean, VA 22102
(703) 821-8955

SERVICES: The clearinghouse was established in 1980 to provide information and educational materials on Sudden Infant Death Syndrome (SIDS). It maintains a library of standard reference materials covering etiology, epidemiology, research, counseling, effects on families, legal aspects, training of emergency personnel, treatment, and prevention of SIDS. The clearinghouse responds to questions, has compiled an annotated research bibliography, and is maintaining and updating mailing lists of state programs, groups, and individuals involved with SIDS. It is a service of the Division of Maternal and Child Health (87-039).

DATABASE: The clearinghouse maintains a computerized in-house Sudden Infant Death Syndrome Database of bibliographic references to patient- and family-oriented print and audiovisual materials. Access is through the clearinghouse.

PUBLICATIONS: Materials are available on sudden infant death syndrome, death and dying, and bereavement. *Information Exchange* (quarterly newsletter).

CLINICAL MEDICINE

87-046 BROOKE ARMY MEDICAL CENTER
MEDICAL LIBRARY
Department of the Army
Health Services Command
Fort Sam Houston, TX 78234
(512) 221-4119 and 221-7182

SERVICES: The library's principal areas of interest are clinical medicine of all health sciences and related fields, with emphasis on patient care, medical research, burns, dentistry, kidneys, nutrition, nursing, and psychiatry.   The library answers inquiries and provides referral, reference, and interlibrary loan services.   It primarily serves Medical Center personnel but, as resources permit, also serves other professional health service personnel.

PUBLICATIONS: Reports of the Brooke Army Medical Center are available from the National Technical Information Service, Springfield, VA 22161.

87-047 FITZSIMONS ARMY MEDICAL CENTER
MEDICAL LIBRARY
Department of the Army
Health Services Command
Bldg. 511
Aurora, CO 80045-5000
(303) 361-8918 and 361-8790

SERVICES: This teaching hospital library specializes in clinical medicine and related sciences, patient administration, clinics, research, and education.   It answers inquiries and provides referral, reference, and interlibrary loan services. The library primarily serves Medical Center staff but, as resources permit, also serves other professional health service personnel.

PUBLICATIONS: The center issues reports based on clinical research investigations; these reports are available from the library on interlibrary loan.

**87-048 LETTERMAN ARMY MEDICAL CENTER
MEDICAL LIBRARY**
Department of the Army
Health Services Command
Bldg. 1100, Rm. 338
Presidio of San Francisco
San Francisco, CA 94129-6700
(415) 561-2465 and 561-3124

SERVICES: The medical library's primary areas of interest are medicine and all of its specialities and subspecialties, medical engineering, hospital administration, and biomechanics. It maintains a large collection of medical journals and a military medical history collection. The library also has access to all National Library of Medicine computerized databases, subscribes to the DIALOG, BRS, and OCLC computerized databases, and is a member of the Pacific Southwest Regional Medical Library Service. It answers inquiries; provides advisory, reference, and literature-searching services; makes referrals to other sources of information; and permits on-site use of its collections. Services are free and are available to physicians and research workers on a referral basis from other information specialists or librarians and to retired military personnel.

**87-049 MADIGAN ARMY MEDICAL CENTER (MAMC)
MEDICAL TECHNICAL LIBRARY**
Department of the Army
Health Services Command
P.O. Box 375

Tacoma, WA 98431-5375
(206) 967-6782 and 967-6298

SERVICES: The MAMC Medical Technical Library emphasizes clinical medicine and surgery. Additional subject areas are
dentistry, nursing, and hospital administration. The library answers inquiries and provides referral, reference, and interlibrary
loan services. It primarily serves Medical Center staff but, as
resources permit, also serves other professional health service
personnel.

PUBLICATIONS: MAMC's *Annual Report,* as well as other
reports covering results of medical studies, are available from the
National Technical Information Service, Springfield, VA 22161.

**87-050 MALCOLM GROW USAF MEDICAL CENTER
MEDICAL LIBRARY**
Department of the Air Force
Andrews Air Force Base
P.O. Box 3097
Washington, DC 20331-5300
(301) 981-2354

SERVICES: The library's areas of interest include medicine,
dentistry, periodontics, prosthodontics, hospital administration,
dietetics, forensic medicine, dermatology, radiology, cardiopul-
monary diseases, veterinary sciences, biochemistry, social work,
psychiatry, laboratory technician training, midwifery, nursing,
and family practice. It answers inquiries; provides advisory,
reference, literature-searching, and reproduction services; makes
interlibrary loans; makes referrals to other sources of information; and permits on-site use of its collections. Services are free
and are available primarily to the center's staff, but others may
use the services by special arrangement with the librarian.

**87-051 WALTER REED ARMY MEDICAL CENTER
MEDICAL LIBRARY**

Department of the Army
Health Services Command
Bldg. 2, Rm. 2-G
Washington, DC 20307-5001
(212) 576-1238

SERVICES: The medical library's areas of interest are clinical medicine, dentistry, nursing, psychiatry, allied health disciplines, military medicine, and the history of military medicine. Its comprehensive collection also includes the Ainsworth Endowment Library of more than 1,000 volumes on the history of military medicine. The library provides reference services to members of the Walter Reed Army Medical Center staff and makes interlibrary loans.

87-052   **WARREN GRANT MAGNUSON CLINICAL CENTER**
Office of Clinical Center Communications
Department of Health and Human Services
National Institutes of Health
Bldg. 10, Rm. 1C-255
9000 Rockville Pike
Bethesda, MD 20892
(301) 496-2563
(301) 496-4891 (Patient Referral)

SERVICES: The clinical center, established in 1953 as the research hospital of the National Institutes of Health (NIH), is designed to bring patient care facilities close to research laboratories so that new findings of basic and clinical scientists can be quickly applied to the treatment of patients. On referral by physicians, patients are admitted to NIH clinical studies on cancer; allergy and infectious diseases; arthritis, diabetes, kidney, and digestive diseases; child health and human development; dental disorders; diseases of the eyes; heart, lung, and blood diseases; neurological and communicative diseases and stroke; and mental and emotional illnesses. The center also serves as a training center for physicians and medical students.

DATABASE: Information on current clinical studies at NIH can also be obtained from the NATIONAL LIBRARY OF MEDICINE/NATIONAL INSTITUTES OF HEALTH INFORMATION SERVICE (87-055). This online service, an electronic bulletin board for health professionals, is available via MINET (MEDICAL INFORMATION NETWORK), a service of the American Medical Association and GTE Telenet.

PUBLICATIONS: Consumer materials are available on volunteer patient programs and admission procedures. The booklet and audiovisual series, *Medicine for the Layman,* covers a wide range of topics including allergies, arthritis, blood transfusions, the brain, cancer, depression, environmental health, epilepsy, heart disease, the lungs, and radiation therapy. Professional materials are available on clinical studies, research, and fellowships. *Clinical Electives for Medical and Dental Students* (annual); *Medical Staff Fellowship Program* (annual); *Training for Careers in Biomedical Research* (annual); and *Current Clinical Studies* (annual). Single copies of publications are available free on request. A publications list is available.

**87-053   WILFORD HALL USAF MEDICAL CENTER
MEDICAL LIBRARY**
Department of the Air Force
Air Training Command
Bldg. 4550
Lackland Air Force Base, TX 78236
(512) 670-7204

SERVICES: The library's areas of interest include medicine, pediatrics, obstetrics and gynecology, orthopedics, pathology, surgery, dentistry, mental health, radiology, veterinary medicine, physical and occupational therapy, nursing, and hospital administration. It answers inquiries; provides advisory, reference, and literature-searching services; makes interlibrary loans; and makes referrals to other sources of information. Services are free, primarily for center staff, but others will be assisted within limits of time and staff.

HOLDINGS: The library's holdings consist of more than 26,000 books and bound volumes of periodicals and some 880 current periodical subscriptions.

COMMUNITY HEALTH CENTERS

**87-054 BUREAU OF HEALTH CARE DELIVERY AND
ASSISTANCE (BHCDA)
COMMUNITY HEALTH CENTERS PROGRAM**
Department of Health and Human Services
Health Resources and Services Administration
Parklawn Bldg., Rm. 7A-55
5600 Fishers Lane
Rockville, MD 20857
(301) 443-2260

SERVICES: The major objectives of the Community Health Centers Program are to assist states, on request, in becoming ready to assume responsibility for Community Health Centers under the Primary Care Block Grant; to ensure that grant-supported Community Health Centers in medically underserved areas are operating efficiently, providing high-quality and appropriate health care, and complying with all grant conditions before responsibility for them is transferred to the states under the Primary Care Block Grant; and to support Migrant Health Projects. Primary Care Centers (Community Health Centers and Migrant Health Centers) are expected to provide a wide range of services, including preventive health and preventive dental care. They must also be able to meet a set of objective standards for evaluating primary care grantee performance at the service delivery level. The standards are in areas such as financial management, clinical management, assessment of need, involvement of users, and health promotion and disease prevention activities. The program answers inquiries and makes referrals to other sources of information. Services are free, and many publications are available to the public.

COMPREHENSIVE HEALTH INFORMATION
RESOURCES

87-055   NATIONAL LIBRARY OF MEDICINE (NLM)
Department of Health and Human Services
National Institutes of Health
Bldg. 38
8600 Rockville Pike
Bethesda, MD 20894
(301) 496-6308 (Information Officer)
(301) 496-6095 (Reference Desk)
(301) 496-6193 (MEDLARS Management)
(800) 638-8480 (MEDLARS Management)

SERVICES: In support of its mission to collect, preserve, and disseminate biomedical information, the library has assembled one of the largest collections of biomedical literature in the world. Included are more than 3.2 million books, journals, technical reports, and other print and audiovisual materials in 40 biomedical fields, as well as the nation's largest medical history collection. NLM provides computer-based literature retrieval services, interlibrary loan services, programs of grant support for medical libraries, toxicology information services, development of audiovisual materials, and publications. Medical reference questions should be directed to the NLM Reference Desk.

DATABASES: NLM's 21 specialized databases comprising the MEDICAL LITERATURE ANALYSIS AND RETRIEVAL SYSTEM (MEDLARS) and TOXNET (TOXICOLOGY DATA NETWORK) are available through a nationwide network of 2,500 centers at universities, medical schools, hospitals, government agencies, and commercial organizations. Its multiple databases contain some 8.0 million references to journal articles and books in the health sciences published after 1965. A user may search the store of references to produce a list of those pertinent to a specific question. Fact Sheets and Pocket Guides describing the databases are available. A MEDLARS management service desk at NLM is staffed to answer questions about the system.

MEDLINE (MEDLARS ONLINE) contains approximately 800,000 references to biomedical journal articles published in the current and three preceding years. An English abstract, if published with the article, is frequently included. The articles are from 3,000 journals published in the United States and foreign countries. Coverage of previous periods (back to 1966) is provided by BACKFILES, searchable online, that total some 3.5 million references. MEDLINE can also be used to update a search periodically. The search formulation is stored in the computer; each month, when new references are added to the database, the search is processed automatically and the results are mailed to the user from NLM.

BACKFILES (MEDLINE BACKFILES). Five backfiles that contain older MEDLINE references (back to 1966).

TOXLINE (TOXICOLOGY INFORMATION ONLINE) is a bibliographic database covering the pharmacological, biochemical, physiological, environmental, and toxicological effects of drugs and other chemicals. Almost all references in TOXLINE have abstracts and/or indexing terms and Chemical Abstracts Service (CAS) Registry Numbers. The TOXLINE database contains more than 1.7 million recent references, while older information is available in BACKFILES.

CHEMLINE (CHEMICAL DICTIONARY ONLINE) is an online chemical dictionary with more than 700,000 records. It contains chemical names, synonyms, CAS Registry Numbers, molecular formulas, NLM file locators, and limited ring information. By providing synonyms and CAS Registry Numbers, which can significantly increase retrieval, CHEMLINE assists the user in searching other MEDLARS databases. CHEMLINE can also be searched to locate classes of chemical substances.

RTECS (REGISTRY OF TOXIC EFFECTS OF CHEMICAL SUBSTANCES) is an online, interactive version of the National Institute for Occupational Safety and Health's (NIOSH) publication *Registry of Toxic Effects of Chemical Substances,* formerly the *Toxic Substances List.* It contains basic acute and chronic toxicity data for more than 78,000 potentially toxic chemicals. Records include toxicity data, chemical identifiers, exposure standards, and status under various federal regulations and programs. The file, maintained by NIOSH, is compiled annually and can be searched by chemical identifiers, type of effect, or other criteria.

CATLINE (CATALOG ONLINE) contains approximately 600,000 citations of books and serials cataloged at NLM. CATLINE gives medical libraries in the network immediate access to authoritative cataloging information, thus reducing the need for the libraries to do their own original cataloging. Libraries also find this database a useful source of information for ordering books and journals and for providing reference and interlibrary loan services.

SERLINE (SERIALS ONLINE) contains bibliographic information on approximately 60,000 serial titles, including all journals that are on order or cataloged for the NLM collection. For many of these, SERLINE has locator information so the user can determine which U.S. medical libraries own a particular journal. SERLINE is used by librarians to obtain information needed to order journals and to refer interlibrary loan requests.

AVLINE (AUDIOVISUALS ONLINE) contains citations of more than 14,000 audiovisual teaching packages covering a wide range of subject areas in the health sciences and cataloged by NLM since 1975. In some cases, review data such as rating, audience levels, instructional design, specialties, and abstracts are included. Procurement information on titles is provided.

HEALTH PLANNING AND ADMIN (HEALTH PLANNING AND ADMINISTRATION) is produced cooperatively by NLM and the American Hospital Association. It contains more than 300,000 references to literature on health planning, organization, financing, management, manpower, and related subjects. The references are from journals indexed for MEDLINE and *Hospital Literature Index,* selected for their emphasis on health care matters. This database will eventually also contain references to nonserial items such as books and technical reports. Included in the database are selected citations from the HEALTH PLANNING

INFORMATION database (87-108), maintained by the National Health Planning Information Center until November 14, 1986.

HISTLINE (HISTORY OF MEDICINE ONLINE) contains more than 70,000 citations of monographs, journal articles, symposia, congresses, and similar composite publications for the library's annual *Bibliography of the History of Medicine*. Its scope includes the history of medicine and related sciences, professions, individuals, institutions, drugs, and diseases of given chronological periods and geographical areas.

The CANCERLINE System of the National Cancer Institute (NCI) consists of three separate databases, all sponsored by NCI: CANCERLIT, CANCERPROJ, and CLINPROT. CANCERLIT (CANCER LITERATURE) contains approximately 500,000 citations and abstracts of published international literature dealing with all aspects of cancer; it is updated monthly with some 5,000 abstracts. Approximately 80 percent of the literature is selected from an international collection of 3,000 biomedical and scientific journals. Nonserial literature (including books, reports, and meeting abstracts) contributes the remaining 20 percent. Informative abstracts averaging 200 words are included for most selected cancer-related documents. The database includes cancer literature from 1963 forward. Literature available for the period 1963 through 1976 is limited to references that had been selected for *Carcinogenesis Abstracts* and *Cancer Therapy Abstracts*. In 1977, the scope of the database was expanded to include all cancer-related literature, except most single case histories. In 1980, new records began including *MeSH* terms for uniform retrieval, and since January 1985, new records have been indexed with chemical names and CAS Registry/EC Numbers. CANCERPROJ (CANCER RESEARCH PROJECTS) contains approximately 5,000 descriptions of current cancer research projects around the world. This file was reactivated in April 1985 and is expected to grow steadily, with quarterly updating, toward an eventual size of approximately 10,000 records. It contains descriptions of federally and privately supported grants and contracts. Twenty percent of the project descriptions are provided by scientists from outside the United States. The project summaries are usually divided into a statement of the research objective, a description of the experimental approach, and a statement of any progress made to date. CLINPROT (CLINICAL CANCER PROTOCOLS) contains summaries of approximately 5,000 clinical trials of new anticancer agents or treatment modalities. Updated monthly, most of the protocols in CLINPROT are provided by the Division of Cancer Treatment (87-031) of the National Cancer Institute, while the remaining protocols are provided by major U.S. cancer centers or sources outside the United States. Protocol summaries include the objective and an outline of the study, patient entry criteria, dosage schedules, dosage forms, and special study parameters. The name and telephone number of the study group chairman are provided. CLINPROT is designed primarily as a reference tool for clinical oncologists.

PDQ (PHYSICIAN DATA QUERY), another link in the National Cancer Institute's efforts to reduce cancer deaths by one half by the year 2000, is an interactive database sponsored by NCI and maintained by ICIC (87-033) that provides ready access to information on state-of-the-art and investigational cancer treatments. This online information system is designed to more effectively disseminate information on cancer treatment to the medical community. The PDQ database consists of three interlinked files, organized and internally arranged to facilitate interactive searching and retrieval of information by users. These files cover cancer information and treatment, a directory of physicians and organizations that provide cancer care, and active NCI-supported protocols from the CLINPROT file. To each of these approximately 700 research protocol descriptions, NCI has added a list of the institutions where the protocol is being used to treat patients and the name of an oncologist to contact at each institution for information about the protocol. The database is menu-driven, which makes it a "user-friendly" system for individuals who are inexperienced in using computers for online information searching.

BIOETHICSLINE contains citations of documents that discuss ethical questions arising in health care or biomedical research. It is a comprehensive, cross-disciplinary collection of references to print and nonprint materials on bioethical topics. Among the publication types included in the database are journal and newspaper articles, monographs, analytics, court decisions, and

Southeastern/Atlantic Regional Medical Library Services
University of Maryland
Health Sciences Library
111 S. Greene St.
Baltimore, MD 21201
(301) 328-2855
(800) 638-6093

STATES SERVED: Alabama, Florida, Georgia, Maryland, Mississippi, North Carolina, South Carolina, Tennessee, Virginia, West Virginia, the District of Columbia, and the Virgin Islands

Greater Midwest Regional Medical Library Network
University of Illinois at Chicago
Library of the Health Sciences
P.O. Box 7509
Chicago, IL 60680
(312) 996-2464
TELEX: 206243

STATES SERVED: Iowa, Illinois, Indiana, Kentucky, Michigan, Minnesota, North Dakota, Ohio, South Dakota, and Wisconsin

Midcontinental Regional Medical Library Program
University of Nebraska
Medical Center Library
42nd St. and Dewey Ave.
Omaha, NE 68105-1065
(402) 559-4326
(1-800) MED-RML4

STATES SERVED: Colorado, Kansas, Montana, Nebraska, Utah, and Wyoming

ONLINE CENTER for Regions 3, 4, and 5

South Central Regional Medical Library Program
University of Texas
Health Science Center at Dallas
5323 Harry Hines Blvd.
Dallas, TX 75235-9049
(214) 688-2085

STATES SERVED: Arkansas, Louisiana, New Mexico, Oklahoma, and Texas

Pacific Northwest Regional Health Sciences Library Service
University of Washington
Health Sciences Library and Information Center
Seattle, WA 98195
(206) 543-8262

   STATES SERVED: Alaska, Idaho, Montana, Oregon, and Washington

Pacific Southwest Regional Medical Library Service
UCLA Biomedical Library
Center for the Health Sciences (12-077)
10833 Le Conte Ave.
Los Angeles, CA 90024-1798
(213) 825-1200

   STATES SERVED: Arizona, California, Hawaii, Nevada, and U.S.
Territories in the Pacific Basin

   ONLINE CENTER for Regions 6 and 7

CONSUMER INFORMATION AND PROTECTION

87-056 **CENTER FOR DEVICES AND RADIOLOGICAL HEALTH**
Division of Consumer Affairs
Department of Health and Human Services
Food and Drug Administration
Chapman Bldg., Rm. 342
5600 Fishers Lane (HFZ-210)
Rockville, MD 20857
(301) 443-4190

SERVICES: The center was formed in 1983 by merger of the bureaus of Medical Devices and Radiological Health. It conducts a national program designed to control unnecessary exposure of humans to, and ensure the safe use of, potentially hazardous ionizing and nonionizing radiation. It also conducts an electronic product radiation control program and a national program designed to protect the consumer by ensuring that medical devices and diagnostic products intended for human use are safe. The Division of Consumer Affairs is responsible for developing consumer education programs, answering consumer inquiries by telephone or mail on general issues relating to medical devices and radiological health, and informing the public on good health care as it relates to medical devices. The center defines a medical device as "a health care product that does not achieve any of its principal intended purposes by chemical action within or on the body or by being metabolized." Devices are such things as tongue depressors, bandages, thermometers, hearing aids, contact lenses, intrauterine devices (IUDs) and heart pacemakers.
PUBLICATIONS: Consumer materials are available on pregnancy test kits, ultraviolet radiation, x-rays, hearing aids, quack medical devices, IUDs, contact lenses, eyeglass lenses, and other general information on medical devices and radiological health

products. Professional materials include listings of *Federal Register* documents about medical devices and radiological health products.

87-057 CONSUMER INFORMATION CENTER (CIC)
General Services Administration
Pueblo, CO 81009
(303) 948-3334

SERVICES: The center, founded in 1970, encourages federal agencies to develop and release useful consumer information on a wide variety of topics. It publishes a catalog of available materials and updates this listing quarterly; it also provides assistance to governmental agencies for the development of pamphlets. The center sends weekly news releases to newspapers, consumer organizations, and governmental agencies. The major function of the center is to distribute federal agency publications through its distribution center. The center responds to mail orders for publications, with a delivery time of approximately three weeks.
PUBLICATIONS: Consumer materials are available on children's health, food, drugs, medical services, exercise, weight control, and diseases and disorders. *Consumer Information Catalog* (quarterly); a similar catalog in Spanish is issued annually. There is a charge for many publications distributed by the center. A $1.00 handling fee is charged when ordering two or more free publications.

87-058 CONSUMER PRODUCT SAFETY COMMISSION (CPSC)
Office of Information and Public Affairs
5401 Westbard Ave., Rm. 332
Washington, DC 20207
(301) 492-6580
(800) 638-2772

SERVICES: The Consumer Product Safety Commission was established in 1972 to reduce the number of injuries and deaths resulting from the use of consumer products. The commission sponsors a toll-free telephone hotline Monday through Friday, 8:30 a.m. to 5:00 p.m., EST, to answer questions about product safety and to receive reports on product-related accidents. CPSC maintains the National Injury Information Clearinghouse (87- 063), conducts research into accidents resulting from consumer products, and establishes product safety standards. The commission assists consumers in evaluating the comparative safety of products and conducts information and educational programs to increase consumer awareness of dangerous products.

DATABASE: CPSC operates the National Electronic Injury Surveillance System (NEISS), which monitors a statistical sample of hospital emergency rooms for injuries associated with consumer products. The system is made up of four files: (1) coded reports on product-related injuries, (2) accident investigations conducted by staff members, (3) death certificates, and (4) consumer complaints.

PUBLICATIONS: Consumer materials are available on children's products, electrical products, product safety, consumer products, accidents, and federal regulations.

87-059   DEPARTMENT OF HEALTH AND HUMAN SERVICES (DHHS)
OFFICE OF CONSUMER AFFAIRS
Premier Bldg., Rm. 1009
1725 I St., NW
Washington, DC 20201
(202) 634-4140

SERVICES: The DHHS Office of Consumer Affairs (OCA), established in 1964 as the President's Committee on Consumer Interests, is responsible for providing the President and federal agencies with advice and information regarding the interests of American consumers. OCA encourages and assists in developing new consumer programs, makes recommendations to improve federal consumer programs, cooperates with state agencies and voluntary organizations in advancing consumer interests, promotes improved consumer education, recommends legislation and regulations to help consumers, and encourages the exchange of ideas among industry, government, and consumers.

PUBLICATIONS: *Consumer's Resource Handbook* is available free from the Consumer Information Center, Dept. 635H, Pueblo, CO 81009. Public service announcements are also sent to radio stations.

87-060 DIRECTORATE OF MEDICAL MATERIEL
Department of Defense
Defense Logistics Agency
Defense Personnel Support Center
Attn: DPSC-RSTS
2800 S. 20th St.
Philadelphia, PA 19101
(215) 952-2116

SERVICES: The Directorate of Medical Materiel prepares specifications and standards for drugs, biologicals, and reagents; for surgical, optical, x-ray, laboratory, dental, and medical equipment used by the military medical services; and for certain chemical analysis instruments and laboratory equipment and supplies used by various federal civil agencies. It answers inquiries of a technical nature pertaining to items within the directorate's areas of interest.

87-061 FEDERAL TRADE COMMISSION (FTC)
Public Reference Branch
6th St. and Pennsylvania Ave., NW, Rm. 130
Washington, DC 20580
(202) 523-3598

SERVICES: The Federal Trade Commission is an independent federal agency that works to maintain a strongly competitive free enterprise system. The commission investigates consumer complaints, writes trade regulations, develops consumer education programs, and protects consumers from unfair and deceptive business practices. Ten regional FTC offices also collect and investigate consumer complaints. The FTC's consumer protection programs focus on health-related topics such as truth in advertising, product reliability, and business practices of health spas and nursing homes.

PUBLICATIONS: Materials are available on federal legislation, court decisions, eyeglasses, generic drugs, health clubs, laser medicine, and contact lenses. Some publications are available free from the FTC Distribution and Duplication Branch; others are sold by the Superintendent of Documents, U.S. Government Printing Office, Washington, DC 20402 and the National Technical Information Service, Springfield, VA 22161. Some of the consumer materials are available in Spanish. Most publications are available free. A publications list is available on request.

FTC REGIONAL OFFICES

Federal Trade Commission Regional Office
10 Causeway St., Suite 1184
Boston, MA 02222-1073
(617) 565-7240

Federal Trade Commission Regional Office
26 Federal Plz., 27th Fl.
New York, NY 10278
(212) 264-1207

Federal Trade Commission Regional Office
1718 Peachtree St., NW, Suite 1000
Atlanta, GA 30367
(404) 347-4836

Federal Trade Commission Regional Office
Mall Bldg., Suite 500
118 St. Clair Ave.
Cleveland, OH 44114
(216) 522-4207

Federal Trade Commission Regional Office
55 E. Monroe St., Suite 1437
Chicago, IL 60603
(312) 353-4423

Federal Trade Commission Regional Office
8303 Elm Brook Dr.
Dallas, TX 75247
(214) 767-7050

Federal Trade Commission Regional Office
1405 Curtis St., Suite 2900
Denver, CO 80202
(303) 844-2271

Federal Trade Commission Regional Office
11000 Wilshire Blvd., Suite 13209
Los Angeles, CA 90024
(213) 209-7890

Federal Trade Commission Regional Office
901 Market St., Suite 570
San Francisco, CA 94103
(415) 995-5220

Federal Trade Commission Regional Office
Federal Bldg., Suite 286
915 2nd Ave.
Seattle, WA 98714
(206) 442-4656

87-062 **FOOD AND DRUG ADMINISTRATION (FDA)**
OFFICE OF CONSUMER AFFAIRS
Department of Health and Human Services
Parklawn Bldg., Rm. 16-63
5600 Fishers Lane (HFE-88)
Rockville, MD 20857
(301) 443-3170

SERVICES: Charged with the responsibility of handling inquiries for FDA, the Office of Consumer Affairs serves as a clearinghouse for its consumer publications. Approximately 70,000 requests are received each year, primarily in the food and cosmetic areas. Inquiries are referred to appropriate agency offices for reply or are answered by the Office of Consumer Affairs staff, utilizing data from agency offices or agency publications. Most inquiries are received by mail. In addition, the Office of Consumer Affairs has assumed responsibility for responding to requests that had been submitted to the Poison Control Branch (87-166) prior to its being disbanded.

PUBLICATIONS: *FDA Consumer* (monthly journal). A publications list is available.

87-063 NATIONAL INJURY INFORMATION CLEARINGHOUSE
5401 Westbard Ave., Rm. 625
Washington, DC 20207
(301) 492-6424

SERVICES: The clearinghouse, begun in 1973, collects, investigates, analyzes, and disseminates injury data and information relating to the causes and prevention of death, injury, and illness associated with consumer products. Newspaper articles on product-related accidents and reports from selected coroners participating in the Medical Examiners and Coroners Alert Program (MECAP) are collected. Paper and microfilm copies of accident investigations, copies of special reports, and formatted reports from the NEISS database are available. The clearinghouse is operated for the Consumer Product Safety Commission (CPSC) (87-058). Charges are assessed when the cost of servicing a request exceeds a certain amount. Requests of a general nature relating to consumer product safety are referred to CPSC.

DATABASE: Data from the National Electronic Injury Surveillance System (NEISS), maintained by the Consumer Product Safety Commission, is used to respond to inquiries. NEISS is a computerized system that monitors a statistical sample of hospital emergency rooms for injuries associated with consumer products. The system is made up of four files: (1) coded reports on product-related injuries, (2) accident investigations conducted by staff members, (3) death certificates, and (4) consumer complaints.

PUBLICATIONS: Professional materials include statistical data on product-related injuries. *NEISS Data Highlights* (annual statistics).

DENTAL RESEARCH

87-064   ARMY INSTITUTE OF DENTAL RESEARCH
Department of the Army
Health Services Command
Walter Reed Army Medical Center
Bldg. 40
6825 16th St., NW
Washington, DC 20307-5300
(202) 576-3450

SERVICES: The Army Institute of Dental Research conducts research in oral disease, maxillofacial injuries, dental materials, and clinical dentistry. Current programs include nondegradable and biodegradable implant materials, precious metal substitutes, and acceleration of bone wound healing. It provides technical answers, referral services, and interlibrary loans to Department of Defense organizations, other governmental agencies, and medical and educational institutions, subject to material and personnel limitations.

87-065   NATIONAL INSTITUTE OF DENTAL RESEARCH (NIDR)
Information Office
Department of Health and Human Services
National Institutes of Health
Bldg. 31, Rm. 2C-35
9000 Rockville Pike
Bethesda, MD 20892
(301) 496-4261

SERVICES: The National Institute of Dental Research was established in 1948 to improve the dental health of Americans through education and research.

PUBLICATIONS: Consumer materials are available on dental health, fluoride treatment, temporomandibular joint disease, canker sores, periodontal disease, cleft lip, cleft palate, dental sealants, and dental implants. Professional materials are available on health promotion, school fluoride programs, statistics, and radiology. *NIDR Research News* (irregular). Single copies of publications are available free.

87-066   NAVAL DENTAL RESEARCH INSTITUTE
Department of the Navy
Naval Medical Research and Development Command
Naval Training Center
Bldg. 1H
Great Lakes, IL 60088-5259
(312) 688-4678

SERVICES: The Naval Dental Research Institute conducts research in dental problems of oral health in Naval and Marine Corps personnel and in the delivery of dental care. Its areas of major interest are dentistry, preventive dentistry, dental caries, dental plaque, dental personnel, oral diseases, oral hygiene, teeth, fluorides, mouth, prophylaxis, histology, pathology, and biochemistry. It provides information service support to Naval organizations, to other Department of Defense organizations, and to members of the Lake County, Illinois Consortium. In addition, it answers queries and provides referral service to others, subject to its facility and personnel limitations.

PUBLICATIONS: The institutes's technical reports are available from the National Technical Information Service, Springfield, VA 22161.

DISEASE PREVENTION

**87-067   OFFICE OF DISEASE PREVENTION AND HEALTH
PROMOTION (ODPHP)**
Department of Health and Human Services
Office of the Assistant Secretary for Health
Mary E. Switzer Bldg., Rm. 2132
330 C St., SW
Washington, DC 20201
(202) 245-7611

SERVICES: The Office of Disease Prevention and Health
Promotion works to promote health and prevent disease among
Americans by overseeing and supporting DHHS initiatives and
programs in prevention. Activities of ODPHP fall into the general categories of policy formulation, coordination, technical assistance, information, and education. Its 1990 Objectives Initiative monitors progress toward the achievement of health objectives for America set forth in *Promoting Health/Preventing
Disease: Objectives for the Nation.* The Nutrition Initiative
works to strengthen the department's leadership in nutrition research services. The Preventive Services Initiative works with
major organizations and institutions toward the delivery of preventive services in health care settings. Initiatives have been in-
stituted to work for health promotion in schools and at worksites.
Media-based efforts to mobilize community resources for health
promotion have contributed to the Community/Media Health
Promotion Initiative. This initiative also includes a thrust for
health promotion for the elderly. ODPHP's Risk Assessment
Review studies the way PHS agencies use quantitative and qual-
itative health risk assessment techniques. ODPHP also operates,
under contract, the ODPHP Health Information Center (87-118)
and the National Information Center on Orphan Drugs and Rare
Diseases (87-159). Inquiries involving matters other than pol-

icy and strategy should be directed to ODPHP, P.O. Box 1133, Washington, DC 20013.

PUBLICATIONS: Materials for professionals are available on federal programs and policy, community and school health promotion programs, health promotion at the worksite, nutrition, and health promotion in health maintenance organizations. Consumer-oriented materials are distributed by ODPHP. Publications must be ordered from ODPHP or the Superintendent of Documents, U.S. Government Printing Office, Washington, DC 20402. A publications list is available from ODPHP.

DRUG ABUSE

87-068 **NATIONAL CLEARINGHOUSE FOR DRUG ABUSE INFORMATION**
P.O. Box 416
Kensington, MD 20795
(301) 443-6500

SERVICES: The clearinghouse, established in 1970, collects, classifies, stores, and disseminates scientific and general information on drug abuse; answers information requests; develops resource materials; and operates the Drug Abuse Communications Network (DRACON), a nationwide linkage of drug information centers affiliated with federal, state, and local governmental agencies, universities, and training centers. The clearinghouse, as a service of the National Institute on Drug Abuse, DHHS, also provides consultation to groups preparing for a seminar, lecture series, panel discussion, or conference to help them assemble the most pertinent and useful materials for the event.

PUBLICATIONS: Consumer materials are available on drugs, drug abuse, prevention, and elderly Americans. Professional materials are available on minority issues, treatment programs, research, and pain. Medical treatment manuals and training guides are also available. A publications list, which is updated bimonthly, may be requested from the clearinghouse.

87-069 **NATIONAL INSTITUTE ON DRUG ABUSE (NIDA) OFFICE OF SCIENCE**
Department of Health and Human Services
Alcohol, Drug Abuse, and Mental Health Administration
Parklawn Bldg., Rm. 10-16
5600 Fishers Lane

Rockville, MD 20857
(301) 443-6480

SERVICES: The major areas of interest of NIDA's Office
of Science are the scientific aspects of drugs of abuse, ranging
from chemistry of abused substances to psychological characteristics of user groups, including biological, behavioral, clinical,
and epidemiological factors in drug abuse. The office answers
inquiries, provides consulting services, and offers limited assistance to individual researchers in the development of grant
applications. Its services are primarily for the scientific community; general inquiries from the public should be directed to the
National Clearinghouse for Drug Abuse Information (87-068).

DATABASES: The Office of Science maintains two in-house
databases: DARPIS (Drug Abuse Research Project Information
System), which contains information about drug abuse research
projects, and RAUS (Research Analysis and Utilization System),
which contains substance abuse research results.

PUBLICATIONS: *Research Monograph Series,* including
RAUS Review Reports (6 to 10 issues a year; publications list
available) and a *Research Issues* series (3 to 4 issues a year).

87-070   NIDA ADDICTION RESEARCH CENTER
Department of Health and Human Services
Alcohol, Drug Abuse, and Mental Health Administration
National Institute on Drug Abuse
Francis Scott Key Medical Center
4940 Eastern Ave., Bldg. C
P.O. Box 5180
Baltimore, MD 21224
(301) 955-7502

SERVICES: The center's main areas of interest are drug addiction, drug abuse, pharmacology, psychopharmacology, neu-
ropharmacology, and neurochemistry. It answers inquiries and
makes interlibrary loans as resources permit.

ENVIRONMENTAL HEALTH AND SAFETY

87-071 ENVIRONMENTAL PROTECTION AGENCY (EPA)
Public Information Center
401 M St., SW (PM-211B)
Washington, DC 20460
(202) 646-6410

SERVICES: EPA's Public Information Center offers a wide variety of information about the agency, its programs and activities, and when appropriate, refers inquirers to the proper technical program or regional office. Other divisions' public information materials on such topics as hazardous wastes, the school asbestos project, air and water pollution, pesticides, and drinking water are distributed through the center. The Public Information Reference Unit provides facilities for public inspection of records supporting agency actions and proposed actions. EPA maintains a headquarters library and libraries in each of its 10 regional offices, which are open to the public. Documents may be used in the libraries, duplicated, or borrowed through interlibrary loan arrangements. The Public Information Center is open to the public during normal working hours, and it will also respond to telephone and mail inquiries.

PUBLICATIONS: Materials are available on air pollution, noise, pesticides, solid waste management, toxic substances, and water pollution.

EPA REGIONAL OFFICES

Environmental Protection Agency
Region 1 Library
JFK Federal Bldg., Rm. 1500
Boston, MA 02203
(617) 565-3298

Environmental Protection Agency
Region 2 Library
26 Federal Plz., Rm. 402
New York, NY 10278
(212) 264-2881

Environmental Protection Agency
Region 3 Library, 3PM21
841 Chestnut St., 5th Fl.
Philadelphia, PA 19107
(215) 597-0580

Environmental Protection Agency
Region 4 Library
345 Courtland St., NE, 1st Fl.
Atlanta, GA 30365-2401
(404) 347-4216

Environmental Protection Agency
Region 5 Library
230 S. Dearborn St., Rm. 1670
Chicago, IL 60604
(312) 353-2022

Environmental Protection Agency
Region 6 Library
1445 Ross Ave., 12th Fl.
Dallas, TX 75272-2733
(214) 655-6444

Environmental Protection Agency
Region 7 Library
726 Minnesota Ave., Rm. L-10
Kansas City, MO 66101
(913) 236-2828

Environmental Protection Agency
Region 8 Library, 8PM-IML
999 18th St., Suite 500
Denver, CO 80202-2413
(303) 293-1444

Environmental Protection Agency
Region 9 Library
215 Fremont St., 6th Fl.
San Francisco, CA 94105
(415) 974-8076

Environmental Protection Agency
Region 10 Library, MD108
1200 6th Ave., 10th Fl.
Seattle, WA 98101
(206) 442-1289

87-072 **NATIONAL INSTITUTE OF ENVIRONMENTAL HEALTH SCIENCES (NIEHS)**
Public Affairs Office
Department of Health and Human Services
National Institutes of Health
P.O. Box 12233
Research Triangle Park, NC 27709
(919) 541-3345

SERVICES: Established in 1966, NIEHS supports and conducts basic research, focusing on the interaction between humans and potentially toxic or harmful agents in the environment. The research concentrates on recognizing, identifying, and investigating environmental factors that may be harmful, and quantifying those factors. NIEHS research also focuses on developing an understanding of the mechanisms of action of toxic agents on biological systems. Information based on research is transmitted to regulatory agencies, other governmental agencies, the Congress, medical and research communities, industry, and the general public. NIEHS research is the basis of preventive programs for environment-related diseases and for action by regulatory agencies. Grants and awards are also made to research organizations.

PUBLICATIONS: Consumer materials are available on environmental health research needs. Professional materials include research reports and directories. *Environmental Health Perspectives* (bimonthly journal).

87-073   **OFFICE OF ENVIRONMENTAL ANALYSIS**
Department of Energy
Office of the Assistant Secretary for Environment,
    Safety, and Health
Forrestal Bldg., Rm. 4G036
1000 Independence Ave., SW
Washington, DC 20545
(202) 586-2061

SERVICES: Activities of the Office of Environmental Analysis, formerly the Environmental Assessments Division, include collecting and coordinating energy-and-the-environment information, including health and safety, related to the impacts associated with all phases of energy production, from extraction of raw materials to power generation and transmission. Areas covered include environmental health and safety acceptability of energy technologies and related research, development, and demonstration; human health effects from energy generation, including occupational health and medical research; health effects research in biological systems; environmental information systems; and assessment of energy technology alternatives, including health, safety, environmental, ecological, social, and economic impacts on local, regional, and national scales. The division answers inquiries, provides information on R&D in progress, distributes publications, and makes referrals to sources within the Department of Energy (DOE) or its contractors. Brief answers are provided free, but charges may be made by contractors for more extensive service. Requests for publications or other technical information on environmental programs may be directed to the DOE Technical Information Center, P.O. Box 62, Oak Ridge, TN 37830, (615) 483-8611, ext. 3-4426.

PUBLICATIONS: Technical reports, journal and conference papers, summaries of ongoing research, other summaries, and overviews.

87-074   **OFFICE OF RADIATION PROGRAMS**
Environmental Protection Agency

Office of the Assistant Administrator for Air and Radiation
NE Waterside Mall, Rm. 708
Washington, DC 20460
(202) 475-9600

SERVICES: The areas of interest of EPA's Office of Radiation Programs are radiological health; health hazards associated with exposure to ionizing and nonionizing radiation; radioactivity; measurement of environmental radiation levels; public health aspects of nuclear energy; technology assessment of nuclear power plants; radiation protection, including the setting of standards and criteria for radiation protection; radioactive waste disposal; natural radiation; development of population dose models; technical assistance to states; and emergency response planning. The office answers inquiries; provides information to state health offices, federal and state agencies, scientific organizations, and industries; and makes referrals to other sources of information.

PUBLICATIONS: The office publishes its findings in appropriate scientific journals and in technical reports of its divisions and laboratories.

87-075   **WALTER REED ARMY MEDICAL CENTER**
HEALTH PHYSICS OFFICE
Department of the Army
Health Services Command
Washington, DC 20307
(301) 427-5107

Located at: Bldg. 188, Forest Glen Section
2681 Linden Lane
Silver Spring, MD 20910

SERVICES: The areas of interest of the Health Physics Office include health physics, protection of personnel and the environment from unwarranted radiation exposure, and radiation hazards. The office answers inquiries; there are no restrictions on information for scientists in related fields, but services for others are limited according to the time and effort required.

ENVIRONMENTAL MEDICINE

87-076 ARMY RESEARCH INSTITUTE OF ENVIRONMENTAL MEDICINE
Department of the Army
Army Medical Research and Development Command
Office of the Surgeon General
Bldg. 42
Kansas St.
Natick, MA 01760-5007
(617) 651-4811

SERVICES: The institute conducts basic and applied research on the effects of heat, cold, high terrestrial elevation, and work and physical fitness on the soldier's performance and health. It serves designers, engineers, and physicians concerned with military performance, casualty prevention, and treatment in extreme climates. The institute answers inquiries and provides referral services subject to material and personnel limitations.

PUBLICATIONS: Reports on research results are available from the National Technical Information Service, Springfield, VA 22161.

87-077 HEALTH EFFECTS RESEARCH LABORATORY
Environmental Protection Agency (MD51)
Office of the Assistant Administrator for Research
and Development
Research Triangle Park, NC 27711
(919) 541-2281

Located at: Alexander Drive and Hwy. 54
Research Triangle Park, NC 27711

SERVICES: The laboratory conducts research to detect, define, and quantify the health effects of environmental pollution. Its primary areas of interest concern the relationships of environmental pollutants, singly or in combination, and their health effects, using toxicological, clinical, and epidemiological studies. The laboratory maintains a collection of scientific publications written by staff members since 1977 and a collection of data resulting from a review of existing literature on selected bioassays for detecting mutagenicity and presumptive carcinogenicity. The laboratory answers inquiries and provides information on research in progress.

PUBLICATIONS: Technical reports and journal articles.

87-078 INFORMATION CENTER FOR INTERNAL EXPOSURE
Oak Ridge National Laboratory
Health and Safety Research Division
Oak Ridge, TN 37830

SERVICES: The center was sponsored by the Division of Biomedical and Environmental Sciences of the Department of Energy. Its areas of interest concerned the estimation of dose received from internally deposited radionuclides, calculation of annual limits on intake of radionuclides, body-burden calculations, and metabolic questions involved in estimating internal exposure. It answered inquiries, conducted literature searches, prepared data compilations, and supplied information and interpretations to the Committees on Internal Dose of the International Commission on Radiological Protection (ICRP) and the National Council on Radiation Protection and Measurement (NCRPM).The Information Center for Internal Exposure was deactivated in late 1986; information it handled is now available from the Toxicology Information Response Center (TIRC), P.O. Box Y, Bldg. 2001, Oak Ridge, TN 37831-6050, (615) 576-1746.

ENVIRONMENTAL TERATOLOGY

**87-079 ENVIRONMENTAL TERATOLOGY INFORMATION
CENTER (ETIC)**
Oak Ridge National Laboratory
Information Research and Analysis Section
Biology Division
Bldg. 9207, MS-3
P.O. Box Y
Oak Ridge, TN 37831
(615) 574-7871

SERVICES: Sponsored by the National Toxicology Program and the Environmental Protection Agency, ETIC collects, organizes, and disseminates information on the testing and evaluation of chemical, biological, and physical agents for teratogenic activity. The center's main areas of interest are information on the testing and evaluation of chemical, biological, and physical agents, and dietary deficiencies for teratological effects in warm-blooded animals. Its main focus is on the administration of an agent to pregnant animals and examination of the offspring at or near birth for structural or functional anomalies. The center provides manual and computerized literature-searching services, makes referrals to other sources of information, and permits on-site use of its hard copy collection. Services are free and available to the public on a mutual information exchange basis as time permits.

DATABASES: ETIC maintains two in-house computerized databases: the Environmental Teratology Information Database is a technically indexed bibliographic file of more than 32,000 references to the literature (journal articles, abstracts, symposia proceedings, books, dissertations, reports, editorials, reviews, methods papers) in the above areas. Chemicals are associated with Chemical Abstracts Service (CAS) Registry Numbers for simplified information retrieval. Hard copy of all references is maintained. The Teratology Data Extraction File contains tabular abstracts of selected articles having specific details pertaining to experimental design, conditions, and observed effects.

PUBLICATIONS: Indexed bibliographies on specific organisms, agents, or test systems (occasionally).

EYE DISORDER RESEARCH

87-080   NATIONAL EYE INSTITUTE (NEI)
Information Office
Department of Health and Human Services
National Institutes of Health
Bldg. 31, Rm. 6A-32
9000 Rockville Pike
Bethesda, MD 20892
(301) 496-5248

SERVICES: NEI, established in 1968, has primary responsibility within the National Institutes of Health and the Federal Government for supporting and conducting research aimed at improving the prevention, diagnosis, and treatment of eye disorders. In addition, NEI encourages the application of research findings to clinical practice, heightens public awareness of eye and vision problems, and cooperates with voluntary organizations that engage in related activities.

PUBLICATIONS: Consumer materials are available on eyes, diabetic retinopathy, low vision, ocular histoplasmosis, retinitis pigmentosa, and senile macular degeneration. Professional materials are available on vision impairment statistics and vision research.

FOOD AND NUTRITION

**87-081   ARMY NATICK RESEARCH, DEVELOPMENT, AND
          ENGINEERING CENTER
          TECHNICAL LIBRARY**
Department of the Army
Army Materiel Command
Bldg. 4
Kansas St.
Natick, MA 01760-5000
(617) 651-4248 and 651-4542

SERVICES: The library's primary areas of interest include
food sciences and engineering, medical science, behavioral sciences, biology, chemistry, clothing, engineering, life sciences,
mathematics, packaging technology, physiology, psychology,
statistics, and textile technology.   Library services are primarily for Natick RD&E Center personnel, but limited access to
open literature collections is available to others by special arrangement.
HOLDINGS: The library's holdings consist of more than
26,500 books, 19,000 bound journals, 1,100 journal subscriptions, and 49,000 technical reports, as well as OCLC computerized systems.
PUBLICATION: The Army Natick Research, Development,
and Engineering Center's *Bibliography of Technical Publications and Papers* (printed annually as a technical report).

87-082   FOOD AND NUTRITION INFORMATION CENTER
Department of Agriculture
National Agricultural Library
Food, Nutrition, and Human Ecology Branch

Rm. 304
Beltsville, MD 20705
(301) 344-3719

SERVICES: Established in 1971 to serve the information needs of persons interested in human nutrition, food service management, and food technology, the center acquires and lends books, journal articles, and audiovisual materials dealing with these areas of concern. The collection ranges from children's books to the most sophisticated professional materials. Books and audiovisual materials may be borrowed from the National Agricultural Library (NAL), and a photoduplication service is available for journal articles. NAL is open to the public from 8:00 a.m. to 4:30 p.m., EST, Monday through Friday. There is a 24-hour answering service to monitor calls for requests during nonbusiness hours.

DATABASE: The center uses the National Agricultural Library's database, AGRICOLA (AGRICULTURAL ON-LINE ACCESS), to do computerized literature searching. AGRICOLA is a bibliographic database that provides access to the worldwide literature on agriculture. Its broad subject scope also highlights food and nutrition. In the United States, it is accessible to the public via DIALOG and BRS.

PUBLICATIONS: Consumer materials include resource guides on various aspects of nutrition, sports, fad diets, hypertension, dental health, elderly Americans, vegetarianism, cancer, diabetes, food composition, anorexia nervosa, bulimia, and alcohol. Professional materials include resource guides on the same topics as the consumer guides, as well as a guide to education and training programs.

87-083 FOOD SAFETY AND INSPECTION SERVICE (FSIS)
Office of Public Awareness
Department of Agriculture
Office of the Assistant Secretary for Marketing and
    Inspection Services
14th St. and Independence Ave., SW, Rm. 1165-S

Washington, DC 20250
(202) 447-9351 (Public Inquiries)
(202) 447-3333 (Meat and Poultry Hotline—Metropolitan
   Washington, DC)
(800) 535-4555 (Meat and Poultry Hotline)

SERVICES: Formerly the Food Safety and Quality Service,
the Food Safety and Inspection Service was established in 1981
to administer the meat and poultry inspection program, which as-
sures consumers that meat and poultry sold in the United States
or shipped abroad is safe, wholesome, and truthfully labeled.
FSIS inspects and analyzes domestic and imported meat, poultry, and meat and poultry food products; establishes standards
and approves recipes and labels for processing meat and poultry products; and monitors the meat and poultry industries for
violations of inspection laws. Questions about meat and poultry
are either answered or referred to the appropriate office.
   PUBLICATIONS: Consumer materials are available on food
safety, food poisoning, poultry products, food additives, meat
products, food labeling, sodium, food inspection, and herbs.
Food News for Consumers (quarterly newsletter). A publications list is available.

87-084   **HUMAN NUTRITION INFORMATION SERVICE (HNIS)**
Department of Agriculture
Office of the Assistant Secretary for Food and
   Consumer Services
Federal Bldg.
6505 Belcrest Rd.
Hyattsville, MD 20782
(301) 436-8617

SERVICES: The Human Nutrition Information Service conducts research in food and nutrition to improve professional and
public understanding of the nutritive value of foods and of the
nutritional adequacy of diets and food supplies. HNIS interprets
the Nationwide Food Consumption Survey and other research re-

sults for the development of food and nutrition guidelines needed by nutrition educators, food program managers, and consumers.

DATABASE: The NUTRIENT DATA BANK is a system maintained by HNIS that contains survey data on nutrient values in foods and descriptions of the foods. It creates for each an average value, which is incorporated into *Agriculture Handbook No. 8, Composition of Foods*. The system operates in batch mode. Although not searchable online, some summarized information from the NUTRIENT DATA BANK can be purchased from the National Technical Information Service, Springfield, VA 22161.

PUBLICATIONS: Consumer materials are available on nutrition and food nutrient values. A list of consumer publications for sale by the Superintendent of Documents, U.S. Government Printing Office, Washington, DC 20402 is available from HNIS. Professional materials are also available on nutrition and food nutrient values. A publications list is available for research workers and teachers.

GENERAL INFORMATION SOURCES

87-085 **FEDERAL INFORMATION CENTER PROGRAM**
General Services Administration
18th and F Sts., NW
Washington, DC 20405
(202) 566-1937

SERVICES: The Federal Information Center (FIC) Program
was established in 1966 as a one-stop source of assistance for
the public about programs and services offered by Federal Government agencies. The most current governmental reference material and service directories, including those in the health area,
are maintained for inquiry research. Second-language ability is
often available. Residents of 72 metropolitan areas can dial an
FIC on a local-call basis; residents of four states may reach an
FIC via a toll-free telephone number. A complete list of FIC
telephone numbers and addresses is available free from the Consumer Information Center, Department 599N, Pueblo, CO 81009
(87-057).

87-086 **LIBRARY OF CONGRESS (LC)**
SCIENCE AND TECHNOLOGY DIVISION
Reference Service
10 1st St., SE, Rm. LA5112
Washington, DC 20540
(202) 287-5687

SERVICES: The Reference Service of LC's Science and
Technology Division provides reference services and is a focal point for the millions of books, journals, and technical re-

ports on scientific and technological topics at the Library of Congress. Direct reference services are provided to users by telephone, mail, or in person at the LC Science Reading Room. Bibliographic guides and research reports by division subject specialists provide indirect reference service. The subject scope of the division includes health-related fields, with the exception of clinical medicine and technical agriculture.

PUBLICATIONS: *LC Science Tracer Bullet* (informal series). Copies of a single *Tracer Bullet* and a master list of the *Tracer Bullet* series are available free from the division. Other materials include health-related titles such as acupuncture, diabetes mellitus, drug abuse, hypertension, birth defects, and medicinal plants. Various library guides are also available.

87-087   **NATIONAL TECHNICAL INFORMATION SERVICE (NTIS)**
Department of Commerce
5285 Port Royal Rd.
Springfield, VA 22161
(703) 487-4600

SERVICES: NTIS was created by Congress in 1950 to provide technical reports and other information products of specialized interest. It is the central source for the public sale of U.S. and foreign government-sponsored research, development, and engineering reports and other analyses prepared by national and local governmental agencies, their contractors and grantees, and other technical groups.

DATABASES: The NTIS Bibliographic Database is searchable online through the commercial vendors DIALOG, BRS, and SDC, or with NTIS assistance. It consists of bibliographic citations or research summaries of the approximately 70,000 technical reports announced annually. The database is updated biweekly and corresponds to the NTIS abstract journal *Government Reports Announcements and Index (GRA&I)*. Surveys indicate the NTIS database is one of the most widely used databases in the world. NTIS also makes available databases from the departments of Energy, Interior, and Agriculture; the National Health

Planning Information Center (87-108); and the National Institutes of Health.

PUBLICATIONS: Materials available include catalogs of services, publications, and computer products in the fields of agriculture and food, biomedical technology and human factors engineering, environmental pollution and control, health planning, medicine and biology, and toxicology.

87-088   U.S. GOVERNMENT PRINTING OFFICE (GPO)
Superintendent of Documents
Washington, DC 20402
(202) 783-3238 (Order Desk)

SERVICES: The U.S. Government Printing Office was founded in 1861 for the production of publications prepared by Congress and agencies and departments of the Federal Government. It was assigned the additional duties of sales and distribution in 1895. Yearly sales today exceed 40 million publications. More than 10,000 different titles may be printed during a single session of Congress.

DATABASE: The GPO PUBLICATIONS REFERENCE FILE is used online at GPO and is accessible to the public through DIALOG and BRS. It contains a complete listing of GPO materials. Searchable fields include subject, title, author, and stock number.

PUBLICATIONS: Materials available include U.S. Government publications; subject bibliographies of publications in more than 250 subject areas are available free. *Health and Health Related Publications* (irregular catalog) is available by free subscription. Except for certain of its catalogs, GPO does not distribute any free publications. Payment is required in advance of shipment; however, single copies of many of its publications are available free from the issuing agencies.

HEALTH AND HUMAN SERVICES PROGRAMS AND EVALUATIONS

87-089 DHHS POLICY INFORMATION CENTER
Department of Health and Human Services
Hubert H. Humphrey Bldg., Rm. 438-F
200 Independence Ave., SW
Washington, DC 20201
(202) 245-6445

SERVICES: Since 1971, the DDHS Policy Information Center, formerly the Evaluation Documentation Center, has identified, collected, and indexed DHHS program evaluations, some in the health area. Also collected are research policy studies in similar areas sponsored by the DHHS Office of the Assistant Secretary for Planning and Evaluation, and studies by the DHHS Inspector General's Office and the General Accounting Office. A one-page description sheet, including an abstract, is prepared for each study. In addition, executive summaries containing problem statements, evaluation objectives, methodology, findings, and recommendations are available for reading at the center; copies of completed studies can be purchased from the National Technical Information Service, Springfield, VA 22161. Inquiries are answered by telephone, mail, or personal assistance.

DATABASE: The center's in-house computerized DHHS Program Evaluation Database provides access to program evaluations by subject and sponsoring agency; custom printouts, including abstracts, are available on request. Sources indexed by this database include 1,600 program evaluation reports. Continual updates add approximately 175 entries annually.

PUBLICATION: *Compendium of HHS Evaluation Studies* (annual).

87-090   OFFICE OF HUMAN DEVELOPMENT SERVICES (OHDS)
Public Affairs Office
Department of Health and Human Services
Hubert H. Humphrey Bldg., Rm. 329-D
200 Independence Ave., SW
Washington, DC 20201
(202) 472-7257

SERVICES: The Public Affairs Office responds to requests
for information on the human services programs administered by
OHDS. OHDS encourages the development of innovative service delivery strategies and works to identify and eliminate, at all
levels of government, barriers to the development of improved
and more accessible social services. Questions are answered
directly or are referred to the appropriate resource.
PUBLICATION: A fact sheet on OHDS is available.

**87-091   OFFICE OF THE ASSISTANT SECRETARY FOR PUBLIC
            AFFAIRS**
Department of Health and Human Services
Hubert H. Humphrey Bldg., Rm. 647-D
200 Independence Ave., SW
Washington, DC 20201
(202) 245-1850

SERVICES: This office's areas of interest cover all aspects
of the department's activities, including public health, medical research, pharmaceuticals, geriatrics, rehabilitation, health
care, social security, and human welfare. It answers inquiries,
provides technical assistance and reference services, evaluates
data, conducts seminars and workshops, distributes DHHS publications, makes referrals to other sources of information, and
permits on-site use of its collection. Services are free and are
available to the public within the limits of the Freedom of Information Act and the Privacy Act.
PUBLICATIONS: A catalog of DHHS publications is available.

87-092 PROJECT SHARE
P.O. Box 2309
Rockville, MD 20852
(301) 231-9539

SERVICES: Established in 1976, Project Share provides reference and referral services, designed to improve the management of human services by emphasizing their integration at the delivery level, to human services planners and managers. In addition, it acquires and makes available to users documents containing current research and development activities, project descriptions, and accounts of the experiences of state and local governments in the planning and management of human services delivery. Access to the collection is achieved through an automated retrieval system. Project Share is a service of the Office of the Assistant Secretary for Planning and Evaluation, DHHS. Fees are charged for publications and selected services.

DATABASE: The Project Share Database is an in-house computerized file of current research and development activities, project descriptions, and accounts of the experiences of state and local governments in the planning and management of human services delivery. Access to the database is through Project Share. The file contains approximately 12,000 records, is updated quarterly, and covers the years since 1972. Abstracts are included for each record, and indexing is done using a taxonomy.

PUBLICATIONS: Professional materials are available on human services administration, program evaluation, elderly board and care, respite care, volunteerism, and domestic violence. *Journal of Human Services Abstracts* (quarterly); *Sharing* (bimonthly newsletter).

HEALTH BENEFIT PROGRAMS FOR FEDERAL
GOVERNMENT PERSONNEL

87-093   **CIVILIAN HEALTH AND MEDICAL PROGRAM OF
          THE UNIFORMED SERVICES (CHAMPUS)**
          Department of Defense
          Office of the Assistant Secretary for Health Affairs
          Aurora, CO 80045-6900
          (303) 361-8606

          Located at: Fitzsimons Army Medical Center
                        Aurora, CO 80045-5000

          SERVICES: CHAMPUS is a health care delivery system of
          the Uniformed Services Health Benefits Program. Spouses and
          children of active duty members of the uniformed services, some
          former spouses, retirees and their family members, and spouses
          and children of deceased active duty members or deceased re-
          tirees have the benefit of coverage under CHAMPUS. Infor-
          mation about CHAMPUS eligibility, benefits, and exclusions is
          available from the Office of CHAMPUS or the health benefits
          advisor at any uniformed services installation.
          PUBLICATIONS: Consumer materials are available on mili-
          tary health benefits and CHAMPUS.

87-094   **OFFICE OF PERSONNEL MANAGEMENT (OPM)**
          Compensation Group
          1900 E St., NW
          Washington, DC 20415
          (202) 632-5582

SERVICES: OPM's areas of interest are benefits payable under the Civil Service Retirement Act; federal employees life insurance and health benefits, and contracts with the carriers; and pay, leave, and hours of duty for federal service. It answers inquiries or refers inquirers to other sources of information and provides consulting and advisory services to governmental agencies.

HEALTH CARE DELIVERY AND ASSISTANCE

**87-095   BUREAU OF HEALTH CARE DELIVERY AND
ASSISTANCE (BHCDA)**
Department of Health and Human Services
Health Resources and Services Administration
Parklawn Bldg., Rm. 705
5600 Fishers Lane
Rockville, MD 20857
(301) 443-2320

SERVICES: Formerly the Bureau of Community Health Services, BHCDA serves as a national focus for efforts to ensure delivery of health care services to residents of medically underserved areas and to special groups. The bureau assists states in providing health care to underserved populations through community health centers and by supporting programs for mothers and children through the Maternal and Child Health Services Block Grant. Funds are provided through project grants to help state, local, voluntary, public, and private entities meet the health needs of special populations such as migrant workers and black lung disease victims. BHCDA provides support for the Bureau of Prisons medical program, a national Hansen's disease program, and the Federal Employee Occupational Health program. It administers a health benefits program for designated Public Health Service beneficiaries and for the National Health Service Corps, which helps states and communities in arranging for physicians, dentists, and other health professionals to provide care in health manpower shortage areas. Inquiries and publication requests are referred to the appropriate BHCDA office for response.

PUBLICATIONS: Publications distributed by BHCDA are listed in the *Health Resources and Services Administration Catalog of Current Publications.* The catalog is available from HRSA's Office of Communications (87-119).

HEALTH CARE FACILITIES

87-096 OFFICE OF HEALTH FACILITIES (OHF)
Department of Health and Human Services
Health Resources and Services Administration
Bureau of Resources Development
Parklawn Bldg., Rm. 11-03
5600 Fishers Lane
Rockville, MD 20857
(301) 443-2086 (Public Affairs Office)
(800) 638-0742 (Toll-free Hotline)
(800) 492-0359 (Maryland Residents)

SERVICES: The Office of Health Facilities was established in October 1982. The scope of activities of its four divisions includes serving as the federal focus for examining capital and financial issues involved in health facilities, administering insured and guaranteed loan programs for health facilities, and monitoring health facilities to determine compliance with assurances made during application for federal construction assistance. OHF also answers questions on the Hill-Burton Free Health Care Program and responds to patient complaints on Hill-Burton facilities via a toll-free hotline. It also answers inquiries, conducts seminars and workshops, and makes referrals to other sources of information. Services are free.

DATABASES: OHF maintains a computerized in-house Health Facilities Database that contains information on facilities obligated under the 20-year uncompensated care assurances program. The data captured for facility obligations begun after January 1959 include location, name, type of facility, date uncompensated service obligation expires, and Hill-Burton grant funds. Another computerized in-house database is the Loan Early Warning System (LEWS), which uses key financial indicators to signal potential financial difficulties of facilities in receipt of DHHS direct and guaranteed loans and FHA-2442 insured loans. LEWS can also be used to examine the fiscal stability of loan applicants. Queries should be addressed to OHF.

PUBLICATIONS: Materials are available on capital formation in health care facilities, cost containment in hospitals through energy conservation, minimum requirements of construction and equipment for hospital and medical facilities, criteria for design review and licensure surveys of solar systems in health care facilities, and energy issues in health facilities.

HEALTH CARE FINANCING

87-097   HEALTH CARE FINANCING ADMINISTRATION (HCFA)
News and Information Branch
Department of Health and Human Services
Hubert H. Humphrey Bldg., Rm. 428-H
200 Independence Ave., SW
Washington, DC 20201
(202) 245-6145

SERVICES: HCFA administers Medicare, Medicaid, and related quality assurance programs. It also makes certain that its beneficiaries are aware of the services for which they are eligible, that services are accessible, and that these services are provided in an effective manner. HCFA ensures that its policies and actions promote efficiency and quality within the total health care delivery system. Questions concerning Medicare or Medicaid can be asked by calling the above number or can be mailed to the agency. Questions are answered or referred to the appropriate office for response. Information on reimbursement programs for kidney dialysis are referred to the appropriate office.

PUBLICATIONS: Consumer materials include descriptive brochures on the Medicare and Medicaid programs and are distributed by local Social Security offices. Professional materials are available on Medicare program statistics, Medicaid program statistics, DRGs (Diagnosis-Related Groups), health care financing, and medical care utilization. *Health Care Financing Review* (quarterly journal).

HEALTH CARE STUDIES

**87-098 HEALTH CARE STUDIES AND CLINICAL
INVESTIGATION ACTIVITY**
Department of the Army
Health Services Command
Bldg. 2268
Fort Sam Houston, TX 78234-6060
(512) 221-4541

SERVICES: The primary areas of interest of this organization
cover all aspects of current developments in (1) health care delivery systems, including quality of care reviews, productivity
evaluations, cost-benefit analyses, ambulatory health care systems, management techniques, medical information systems, and
ancillary medical personnel; (2) nursing systems, nurse clini-
cians, and nurses in federal services; (3) social and behavioral
sciences, including social work, psychology, psychiatry, organizational development, consultation, innovation, human relations
training, systems theory, and attitudinal and satisfaction studies;
(4) dental care delivery systems, including dental epidemiology,
dental program evaluation, dental reporting systems, dental auxiliaries, and military dental development; and (5) monitoring of
all inquiries concerning clinical health problems, institutional review board activities, and protection of human subjects requirements.   It answers inquiries, provides advisory and reference
services, lends materials, distributes copies of reports, and permits on-site use of its collection. Services are free and primarily
for Army medical personnel, but others will be assisted as time
and resources permit.

HEALTH LEGISLATION AND RELATED STUDIES

87-099 CONGRESSIONAL LEGISLATIVE STATUS OFFICE
Congress of the United States
House Office Bldg.
Annex 2, Rm. 696
Washington, DC 20515
(202) 225-1772

SERVICES: This office provides information on the status of
health legislation in either the House or Senate, whether committee hearings have been held, and dates of upcoming meetings.

87-100 GENERAL ACCOUNTING OFFICE (GAO)
Information Office
441 G St., NW
Washington, DC 20548
(202) 275-2812

SERVICES: GAO assists Congress in carrying out its legislative and oversight responsibilities and makes recommendations
designed to provide for more efficient and effective governmental operations.
PUBLICATIONS: There are a number of significant reports in
the health and health care areas. A monthly listing of reports
issued by GAO is available.

87-101 HOUSE DOCUMENT ROOM
U.S. House of Representatives
U.S. Capitol, Rm. H-226
Washington, DC 20515
(202) 225-3456

SERVICES: The House Document Room provides information on the availability of House bills, reports, and public laws. All House documents must now be obtained from the Senate Document Room (87-103).

87-102 OFFICE OF TECHNOLOGY ASSESSMENT (OTA)
Health Program
Congress of the United States
600 Pennsylvania Ave., SE
Washington, DC 20510
(202) 226-2070
(202) 224-8966 (Publications)

SERVICES: OTA assesses complex scientific and technological issues for the benefit of congressional committees. Comprehensive analyses are conducted on issues such as energy, the environment, national security, transportation, and health. It provides reports, testimony, and workshops to clarify the range of policy options on a specific issue and the potential effects of adopting each option.

PUBLICATIONS: Materials are available on the cost-effectiveness of medical technology, the federal immunization policy, food contaminants, physician supply, medical information systems, the effects of proposed changes in health insurance programs on medical technology, priorities for tropical disease research, aging, genetic therapy, occupational health, medical devices, pharmaceuticals, health care costs, the handicapped, and environmental health. *Abstracts of Case Studies in the Health Technology Case Study Series* (monthly). The research reports are for sale by the National Technical Information Service, Springfield, VA 22161, or the Superintendent of Documents, U.S. Government Printing Office, Washington, DC 20402. Availability and price information can be obtained from OTA. Report summaries and abstracts are available to the public free of charge. A publications list and an informational brochure are also available.

87-103   SENATE DOCUMENT ROOM
U.S. Senate
Hart Senate Office Bldg., Rm. B-04
Constitution Ave. and 2nd St., NE
Washington, DC 20510
(202) 224-7860

SERVICES: The Senate Document Room provides information on the availability, and/or copies, of Senate and House bills, reports, and public laws.

87-104   SENATE SPECIAL COMMITTEE ON AGING
Hart Senate Office Bldg., Rm. 628
Constitution Ave. and 2nd St., NE
Washington, DC 20510
(202) 224-5366

SERVICES: This committee is concerned with the problems and opportunities of the elderly, including health, employment, retirement income, housing, and medical and social services. In response to queries, the committee provides information on federal legislation related to aging.
PUBLICATIONS: Reports and transcripts of hearings, staff reports, newsletters, information papers, legislative and budget analyses, and an annual report (a comprehensive review of federal programs and policies).

HEALTH MAINTENANCE ORGANIZATIONS

87-105 OFFICE OF PREPAID HEALTH CARE
Department of Health and Human Services
Health Care Financing Administration
North Bldg., Rm. 4360
330 Independence Ave., SW
Washington, DC 20201
(202) 245-0815

SERVICES: The Office of Prepaid Health Care, formerly the
Office of Health Maintenance Organizations (HMOs), fosters
the development of organized systems of health care for de-
livering comprehensive medical services to voluntarily enrolled
populations on a prepaid capitation basis. It acts as a national
clearinghouse for prepaid health care information and answers
queries or refers them to other sources of information.

PUBLICATIONS: *HMO Act of 1973, P.L. 93-222, as
Amended;* all current HMO regulations; *Prospectus on Health
Maintenance Organizations; Annual Report to the Congress:
Health Maintenance Organizations; Employer Attitudes Toward
HMOs; Investors Guide to Health Maintenance Organizations;
Community Education Tips for HMO Sponsors; Employers,
HMOs, and Dual Choice; A Business Perspective on HMOs;
Guide to Starting a Community Sponsored HMO; Address List
of Operational HMOs in the United States; Planning Medical
Equipment for HMOs; Questions Physicians Ask About HMOs;*
bibliographies; fact sheets; and cost savings sheets.

HEALTH OCCUPATION STATISTICS

**87-106   OFFICE OF ECONOMIC GROWTH AND EMPLOYMENT
            PROJECTIONS (OEGEP)**
Department of Labor
Bureau of Labor Statistics
601 D St., NW, Rm. 4000
Washington, DC 20212
(202) 272-5381

SERVICES: OEGEP analyzes occupations in the United
States and develops statistical projections and factual career information. The Bureau of Labor Statistics maintains eight regional offices. Materials are available, for a fee, on various
health careers.

PUBLICATION: Its *Occupational Outlook Handbook,* published every two years, covers several hundred occupations and
describes what the work involves, the training and education
required, earnings, working conditions, related occupations, job
prospects for the decade ahead, and referral groups for additional
information.

HEALTH PLANNING

87-107 **BUREAU OF RESOURCES DEVELOPMENT**
Department of Health and Human Services
Health Resources and Services Administration
5600 Fishers Lane
Rockville, MD 20857

SERVICES: Formerly the Bureau of Health Maintenance Organizations and Resources Development, Office of Health Planning, this office administered a program of federal, state, and areawide health planning and health delivery systems development. The program created a nationwide network of state and local agencies responsible for preparing and implementing plans to improve the health of residents of their respective areas by increasing the accessibility, acceptability, continuity, and quality of health services in the areas and by restraining increases in the costs of health services. The bureau's health planning program was discontinued on November 14, 1986. Copies of health planning reports can be purchased from the National Technical Information Service, Springfield, VA 22161. Online access to computerized information describing the health planning literature is available by searching the NTIS database (87-087) and the HEALTH PLANNING AND ADMIN database (87-055) of the National Library of Medicine.

87-108 **NATIONAL HEALTH PLANNING INFORMATION**
     CENTER (NHPIC)
Department of Health and Human Services
Bureau of Resources Development
5600 Fishers Lane
Rockville, MD 20857

SERVICES: The center was created to provide information for use in the analysis of issues and problems related to health planning and health care resources development. Reference service and referrals to other information centers were provided. NHPIC maintained microfiche depositories of noncopyrighted health planning reports at 10 locations throughout the United States. The center was discontinued on November 14, 1986.

DATABASE: The online HEALTH PLANNING INFORMATION database contains citations of approximately 27,000 documents. Searches for NHPIC documents can be done through the NTIS database (87-087). In addition, a portion of the health planning database is accessible through the HEALTH PLANNING AND ADMIN file (87-055), a specialized MEDLARS database of the National Library of Medicine.

PUBLICATIONS: *Health Planning and Health Services Research* and *Health Planning Information* (irregular monographs). Other serial publications focused on international activities and case studies in health planning. Copies of NHPIC publications are available from the National Technical Information Service, Springfield, VA 22161.

HEALTH PROFESSION EDUCATION AND TRAINING

87-109   BUREAU OF HEALTH PROFESSIONS
DIVISION OF ASSOCIATED AND DENTAL HEALTH
** PROFESSIONS**
Department of Health and Human Services
Health Resources and Services Administration
Parklawn Bldg., Rm. 8-101
5600 Fishers Lane
Rockville, MD 20857
(301) 443-6853

SERVICES: The Division of Associated and Dental Health
Professions serves as a principal focus with regard to health
professions education, practice, and service research in the fields
of dentistry, optometry, pharmacy, veterinary medicine, public
health, health administration, and allied health professions and
occupations, including dental hygienists, expanded function dental auxiliaries, dental assistants, and dental technicians. It supports and conducts programs, surveys, and studies to analyze
and improve the quality, development, organization, utilization,
and credentialing of personnel in these fields. It also supports
and conducts special educational initiatives to improve the nation's capacity to respond in areas related to health promotion
and disease prevention, nutrition, long-term care and geriatrics,
dental care, and other personnel-related health service delivery
and environmental health and hazard control issues.

PUBLICATIONS: Professional materials are available on dental care, dental schools, dental manpower, allied health education programs, chiropractic health care, hospices, optometry,
health professionals credentialing, and speech-language-hearing
personnel. A publications list is available.

87-110   **BUREAU OF HEALTH PROFESSIONS**
         INFORMATION OFFICE
         Department of Health and Human Services
         Health Resources and Services Administration
         Parklawn Bldg., Rm. 8A-03
         5600 Fishers Lane
         Rockville, MD 20857
         (301) 443-2060

SERVICES: The bureau, formerly the Bureau of Health Manpower, supports development of the human resources needed to staff the U.S. health care system. It is concerned with health professions education, credentialing of health care personnel, and analysis of data to project needs for health professions personnel. Strategies used to achieve these objectives include institutional support; student assistance; analysis of current and future personnel supply, requirements, and distribution; and targeted programs to increase the force of primary care practitioners and to improve the geographic and specialty distribution of health personnel. The bureau provides financial support to institutions for the development of health professionals by targeting resources to areas of high national priority such as disease prevention, health promotion, care of the elderly, and bedside nursing. It also provides financial support to individuals, assuring access to health careers for the disadvantaged. The bureau provides technical information services and assistance to the regional offices of the department, to state and local agencies, and to other federal agencies. Limited edition material may be made available to organizations or persons with a special interest in programmatic information for research and analysis purposes. Information on the bureau's activities may also be obtained from the department's regional offices. Inquiries should be directed to the Regional Health Administrator, DHHS, at the nearest regional office.

PUBLICATIONS: Materials are available on health care databases, health professions education, and health manpower. Booklets, leaflets, and fact sheets that include explanatory program material and information of general public interest are made available in response to inquiries.

**87-111 NATIONAL LIBRARY OF MEDICINE (NLM)
AUDIOVISUAL RESOURCES SECTION (AVRS)**
Department of Health and Human Services
National Institutes of Health
Bldg. 38, Rm. 1W-20
8600 Rockville Pike
Bethesda, MD 20894
(301) 496-4244

SERVICES: The mission of AVRS is to (1) conduct a program to increase the availability of effective instructional media and related learning resources to health professionals, schools, and organizations; (2) release announcements and provide information about available materials; (3) identify instructional materials suitable for sale, loan, or duplication and arrange for their entry into the distribution system; (4) manage a distribution system for instructional materials in the health sciences, including sales, loan, and duplication services; (5) support a program for the review and preservation of 16mm films of significant historical value in the health sciences; (6) develop and manage the NLM Learning Resource Center, which is to serve as a national model for the professional media needs of health professionals, scientists, scholars, students, and paramedical personnel working in programs of national and international significance; and (7) maintain a collection of approximately 5,000 3/4-inch videocassette titles and some 1,000 historical films. Most audiovisual loans must be requested through interlibrary loans.

DATABASE: AVLINE (AUDIOVISUALS ONLINE) is an online database that contains bibliographic citations to more than 14,000 teaching packages, available on loan from AVRS, covering subject areas in the health sciences and cataloged by NLM since 1975. In some cases, review data such as rating, audience levels, instructional design, specialties, and abstracts are included. Procurement information on titles is provided. One of NLM's specialized databases, AVLINE is accessible to the public through MEDLARS.

PUBLICATIONS: *NLM Audiovisuals Catalog* (quarterly); *Health Sciences Audiovisuals* (quarterly microfiche of AVLINE database).

87-112 NAVAL HEALTH SCIENCES EDUCATION AND
TRAINING COMMAND
INSTRUCTIONAL PROGRAMS DIVISION
Department of the Navy
Naval Medical Command
Bethesda, MD 20814-5022
(202) 295-1390

SERVICES: The Instructional Programs Division develops
and manages instructional programs related to health and allied health education, paramedical occupations, military health
occupations, alcohol and drug education, clinical experiences,
and first aid. It maintains a collection of curriculum outlines
(unit/lesson topic titles and objectives) for various allied health
instructional programs conducted by the Naval Medical Command, as well as Medical Department correspondence courses.
The division answers inquiries, provides advisory services, conducts seminars and workshops, lends materials, and permits on-
site use of its collection. Services are available to any nonprofit,
publicly funded programs; some are free and some may be provided for a fee.

87-113 VETERANS ADMINISTRATION (VA)
CENTRAL OFFICE FILM LIBRARY (037B1)
Department of Administrative Services
810 Vermont Ave., NW
Washington, DC 20420
(202) 233-2793

SERVICES: The library maintains an extensive collection of
motion picture films, filmstrips, slides, and audio and video cas-
settes for use in support of medical and scientific research programs and studies and for orientation, training, and information.
It lends films free on receipt of VA Form 3-3785, "Request for
Films."
PUBLICATION: *VA Film Catalog.*

**87-114 VETERANS ADMINISTRATION (VA)
MEDICAL MEDIA PRODUCTION SERVICE**
Veterans Administration Hospital
1030 Jefferson Ave.
Memphis, TN 38104
(901) 577-7279

SERVICES: The VA Medical Media Production Service provides hospital staff members with complete illustration services for records, publications, research, and education. The medical illustrations, both art and photographic, depict abnormal and typical aspects of diseases. The service maintains a library of approximately 250,000 slides of abnormal pathological conditions in patients, cross-referenced by diagnosis. The collection is available to qualified VA staff members, related teaching schools, and cooperating physicians and scientists. Consulting services on biological and medical illustration problems are available to the VA staff.

HEALTH PROMOTION AND EDUCATION

**87-115   CENTER FOR HEALTH PROMOTION AND EDUCATION
(CHPE)**
Department of Health and Human Services
Centers for Disease Control
1600 Clifton Rd., NE
Atlanta, GA 30333
(404) 329-3942

SERVICES: CHPE, established in October 1980, has four divisions (Health Education, Nutrition, Reproductive Health, and the Office on Smoking and Health) and, in its Office of the Director, the Educational Resources Branch. The center offers technical assistance and expertise in these categorical areas and in health promotion and health education. Primary recipients of technical assistance are official state and local health agencies, schools, and health care delivery settings. The Division of Health Education (formerly the Bureau of Health Education, established in 1974) serves as a key resource for health education methodology and programmatic intervention for addressing today's health risks from smoking; nutrition, obesity, and weight management; lack of exercise and physical fitness; hypertension; stress; and alcohol. The center works closely with other federal agencies addressing these topics.

DATABASES: The center maintains a HEALTH EDUCATION database containing information on health education programs in schools, rural and urban communities, medical care facilities and settings, and work environments. The database was established to support CHPE's technical assistance and capacity-building efforts in health promotion and education. The center is developing the AIDS SCHOOL HEALTH EDUCATION database, which contains programs, curricula, guidelines, policies, regulations, and materials. Both databases are part of the COMBINED HEALTH INFORMATION DATABASE (CHID) available online through BRS.

PUBLICATIONS: A variety of publications are produced for professional audiences. *Focal Points* (irregular newsletter).

87-116 NATIONAL AUDIOVISUAL CENTER
Product Acquisition/Marketing Section
National Archives and Records Administration
8700 Edgeworth Dr.
Capital Heights, MD 20743-3701
(301) 763-1850

SERVICES: The National Audiovisual Center is the central source for purchasing or renting the more than 12,000 federally produced audiovisual programs available to the public. Catalogs and referrals to free-loan sources are provided on request. Several of the catalogs cover health-related topics, including such areas as alcohol and drug abuse, dentistry, emergency medical services, industrial safety, medicine, and nursing.

DATABASE: The center maintains an in-house computerized Audiovisual Materials data file containing information on audiovisual materials produced by the Federal Government that are available to the public.

PUBLICATIONS: *Reference List of Audiovisual Materials Produced by the U.S. Government* and other catalogs of available titles are issued and updated on an irregular basis.

87-117 NATIONAL DIFFUSION NETWORK (NDN)
Department of Education
Office of the Assistant Secretary for Educational Research
    and Improvement
Recognition Division
555 New Jersey Ave., NW, Suite 510
Washington, DC 20208
(202) 357-6139

SERVICES: NDN makes educational programs available for adoption by schools, colleges, and other institutions by providing dissemination funds to programs considered to be exemplary. Persons known as facilitators, who serve as matchmakers between schools and NDN programs, are also funded by NDN. Many subject areas are represented among the 99 programs. Several are health related, including programs for physical fitness and drug education. A number of the programs are designed for handicapped persons. More than 18,000 program adoptions were completed in 1982-1983. Services of NDN are oriented to teachers and educational administrators. Persons interested in obtaining more information are directed to contact one of the 55 facilitators. A list of facilitators is available from NDN.

PUBLICATIONS: Professional materials include a list of NDN programs and are available free.

87-118   **ODPHP HEALTH INFORMATION CENTER**
P.O. Box 1133
Washington, DC 20013-1133
(202) 429-9091
(800) 336-4797

SERVICES: The ODPHP Health Information Center, established in 1979 as the National Health Information Clearinghouse, helps the public locate health information through identification of health information resources, an information and referral system, and publications. Utilizing a database that contains descriptions of health-related organizations, center staff refers inquiries to the most appropriate resource. A direct answer is provided primarily to requests for names and addresses of organizations, publication ordering information, inquiries regarding the center, or inquiries for which the staff has no database resource. A core collection of health reference materials, journals, and newsletters is available for use by the public; advance arrangements are recommended. The National Information Center on Orphan Drugs and Rare Diseases (87-159), a component of the center, answers inquiries about rare diseases and orphan products. The center is a service of the Office of Disease Prevention and Health Promotion (ODPHP) (87-067). Center staff will not provide diagnosis or recommend treatment for medical conditions.

DATABASE: The center maintains an internal HEALTH RELATED ORGANIZATIONS database that contains approximately 1,000 descriptions of health information resources such as those maintained by information clearinghouses, technical libraries, professional societies, private foundations, and federal and state agencies. This database has been made available to the National Library of Medicine to be included in the library's online DIRLINE database (87-055), a directory of health information resources based on machine-readable descriptions provided by ODPHP and the former National Referral Center of the Library of Congress. Access to DIRLINE is through MEDLARS. A thesaurus of health information terms is available from the center for a small handling fee. ODPHP'S *Healthfinders,* a series of annotated resource lists on various health topics, are included, full text, in the HEALTH INFORMATION subfile of the COMBINED HEALTH INFORMATION DATABASE (CHID) available through BRS.

PUBLICATIONS: Materials available include resource guides on topics such as medications, health observances, toll-free telephone numbers for health information, stress, vitamins, health statistics, herpes, exercise for the elderly, weight control, health promotion software, health risk appraisals, health fairs, and health care financing. A publications list is available.

HEALTH RESOURCES AND SERVICES

87-119 HEALTH RESOURCES AND SERVICES
ADMINISTRATION (HRSA)
OFFICE OF COMMUNICATIONS
Department of Health and Human Services
Parklawn Bldg., Rm. 14-43
5600 Fishers Lane
Rockville, MD 20857
(301) 443-2086

SERVICES: HRSA's Office of Communications provides information on programs for the distribution, supply, use, quality, and cost-effectiveness of health resources and on health services programs for certain segments of the population. Specific areas of concentration are health professions training, health services for Native Americans and Hansen's disease patients, community health centers, maternal and child health, migrant health, health planning, health facilities, health maintenance organizations, and the National Health Service Corps and scholarship program. Inquiries are either answered directly or referred to the proper bureau or clearinghouse for response.

PUBLICATIONS: Publications include informational material, reports, bibliographies, studies, and guidelines. A catalog of current publications, which includes titles from the bureaus and clearinghouses comprising HRSA, is available.

HEALTH SERVICES RESEARCH AND HEALTH CARE TECHNOLOGY ASSESSMENT

87-120 NATIONAL CENTER FOR HEALTH SERVICES RESEARCH AND HEALTH CARE TECHNOLOGY ASSESSMENT
Department of Health and Human Services
Parklawn Bldg., Rm. 18-12
5600 Fishers Lane
Rockville, MD 20857
(301) 443-4100

SERVICES: The center, established in 1968, is the primary source of federal support for research on problems related to the quality and delivery of health services. It responds to the need for better data and information, new techniques, and innovative methods for improving health care delivery. Center programs evaluate health services, assess technologies, and improve access to new scientific and technical information for research users. Research findings are disseminated through publications, conferences, and workshops. The center maintains a library of its publications and other relevant DHHS publications. Its research is targeted toward the needs of health care policymakers, including executive and legislative officials at federal, state, and local levels; health care administrators; and others with responsibility for health care resource allocations.

PUBLICATIONS: Materials are available on health care costs and utilization, health care expenditures, health information systems, health technology assessment, and grants and contracts. *Health Technology Assessment Reports* (annual); *HCUP Research Notes* (irregular reports); *National Health Care Expenditure Study Data Previews* (irregular); *Hospital Studies Program Research Notes* (irregular); *Long Term Care Studies Program Research Reports* (irregular); *NCHSR Research Activities* (monthly newsletter). Single copies of publications are available free on request from the center (send mailing label). An annotated publications list is also available.

HEALTH STATISTICS

87-121 CLEARINGHOUSE ON HEALTH INDEXES
Department of Health and Human Services
National Center for Health Statistics
Center Bldg., Rm. 2-27
3700 East-West Hwy.
Hyattsville, MD 20782
(301) 436-7035

SERVICES: The clearinghouse provides informational assistance in the development of health measures to health researchers, administrators, and planners. Its definition of a health index is "a measure that summarizes data from two or more components and that purports to reflect the health status of an individual or defined group." Services provided to users include searches of the in-house database, annotated bibliographies, and reference and referral. A library of 4,000 documents and journals is available to users by appointment.

DATABASE: The clearinghouse maintains a computerized in-house Health Index Database to sources such as those found in journal articles, books, conference proceedings, government publications, unpublished materials, speeches, and research in progress. The database is comprehensive since its origin in 1973 and includes coverage of other core materials published earlier.

PUBLICATION: *Bibliography on Health Indexes* (quarterly).

87-122 NATIONAL CENTER FOR HEALTH STATISTICS (NCHS)
Scientific and Technical Information Branch
Department of Health and Human Services
Center Bldg., Rm. 1-57
3700 East-West Hwy.

Hyattsville, MD 20782
(301) 436-8500

SERVICES: Organized in 1960, NCHS has collected, analyzed, and disseminated data on health in the United States. Using surveys and inventories, data systems have been developed to collect statistics on births, deaths, marriages, and divorces in the United States; the extent and impact of illness and disability; determinants of health; health personnel and services; utilization of health care; health care costs and financing; and family growth and dissolution. The center answers requests for data and provides consulting services to foreign, state, and local health officials in the field of health statistics. Staff members respond to requests from professionals or consumers using publications, computer printouts, microdata tapes, and special tabulations. Requests for current statistical information on infectious diseases should be directed to the Centers for Disease Control (87-131) rather than to NCHS.

DATABASE: Much of the data collected and compiled by NCHS is part of the NTIS database (87-087), available online to the public through DIALOG, BRS, and SDC. There is no exclusive NCHS database.

PUBLICATIONS: Materials available include statistical data on health, nutrition, vital statistics, health care delivery, dental health, health resources utilization, health care personnel, families, contraception, and health care economics. *Vital Statistics of the United States* (annual report); *Monthly Vital Statistics Report; Advance Data from the Vital and Health Statistics Series* (irregular); *Statistical Notes for Health Planners* (irregular); *Where to Write for Vital Records: Births, Deaths, Marriages, and Divorces; Health, United States* (annual). A publications list, indexed by subject, is available on request. Most NCHS publications must be purchased from the Superintendent of Documents, U.S. Government Printing Office, Washington, DC 20402. The major reports may be found in large public or university libraries.

**87-123 VETERANS ADMINISTRATION (VA)
BIOMETRICS DIVISION**
810 Vermont Ave., NW
Washington, DC 20420
(202) 233-3458

SERVICES: The principal areas of interest of VA's Biometrics Division are statistical data on VA hospital and nursing home patients since 1970. The data consist of medical and demographic information. Patient data in the files include diagnosis, patient type, length of hospital stay, age, sex (predominantly male), marital status, and state and county of residence. The division responds to inquiries from qualified individuals and organizations involved in biomedical research.

PUBLICATIONS: Several special statistical reports on the VA patient population, for example, *The Most Frequently Occurring Diagnosis in VA Hospitals; Alcoholism and Problem Drinking Among VA Hospital Patients; VA Hospital Patients with Arthritic Conditions;* and *Activities of Daily Living in VA Nursing Home Patients.*

HEART, LUNG, AND BLOOD

**87-124 HIGH BLOOD PRESSURE INFORMATION CENTER
(HBPIC)**
2121 Wisconsin Ave., NW, Suite 410
Washington, DC 20007
(202) 944-3176

SERVICES: The center, which began in 1973, is a source
of informational and educational materials for consumers,
providers, and planners of high blood pressure control services.
Print and audiovisual educational materials are collected from
a variety of sources. Access to information on locations and
services of community programs and activities is also available.
Services of the center include response to inquiries, development
and publication of informational and educational materials, and
distribution of materials from the National High Blood Pressure
Education Program and other organizations. HBPIC is a service
of the National Heart, Lung, and Blood Institute, DHHS.

DATABASE: HBPIC maintains an online HIGH BLOOD PRES-
SURE INFORMATION database that contains more than 4,000
items relating to hypertension, dating from 1973. A thesaurus is
used for indexing and accessing purposes. In January 1985, the
center became a member of the COMBINED HEALTH INFORMA-
TION DATABASE (CHID), available through BRS. The HBPIC file
contains descriptions of more than 600 documents; 20 percent
are directed toward patient audiences and 80 percent are directed
toward professionals.

PUBLICATIONS: Consumer materials are available on high
blood pressure, sodium, and blood pressure measurement devices. Professional materials are available on high blood pressure, worksite programs, community program development, pa-

tient tracking, compliance, patient education, and program evaluation. *Information Memorandum* (bimonthly).

**87-125   LETTERMAN ARMY INSTITUTE OF RESEARCH (LAIR)
HERMAN MEMORIAL LIBRARY**
Department of the Army
Office of the Surgeon General of the Army
Army Medical Research and Development Command
Bldg. 1110, Rm. AS-2302
Presidio of San Francisco
San Francisco, CA 94129-6800
(415) 561-2600 and 561-4767

SERVICES: The library's areas of interest are dermatology research, blood research, laser research, pesticides, and trauma and shock research. The library provides ready reference service and reprints of articles prepared by the LAIR staff, makes interlibrary loans, and permits on-site use of its collection. Services are available to professional personnel, organizations, and teaching institutions.

PUBLICATIONS: *LAIR Reports* and *LAIR Technical Notes* are available from the National Technical Information Service, Springfield, VA 22161.

87-126   NATIONAL HEART, LUNG, AND BLOOD INSTITUTE
Public Inquiries and Reports Branch
Department of Health and Human Services
Bldg. 31, Rm. 4A-21
9000 Rockville Pike
Bethesda, MD 20892
(301) 496-4236

SERVICES: The institute was established in 1948 as the National Heart Institute; in 1976, its name was changed by legislative mandate to the National Heart, Lung, and Blood Institute. The primary responsibility of the institute is the scientific investigation of heart, blood vessel, lung, and blood diseases. The institute oversees research, demonstration, prevention, education, control, and training activities in these fields. Its program emphasizes the prevention and control of heart, lung, and blood diseases, as well as education concerning these diseases, through more rapid transfer of knowledge into the mainstream of clinical medicine and personal health practices.

PUBLICATIONS: Consumer materials are available on Cooley's anemia, exercise, heart disease, the heart, the lungs, arteriosclerosis, congestive heart failure, extrasystoles, cholesterol, hyperlipoproteinemia, pulmonary embolism, high blood pressure, varicose veins, emphysema, chronic obstructive pulmonary disease, smoking, heat stroke, angina, stroke, and blood transfusions. Professional materials are available on arteriosclerosis, blood transfusion, nutrition counseling, lipid research, blood banking, hypertension, fetal hemoglobinopathies, cardiovascular diseases, coronary heart disease, and aplastic anemia. Inquiries should be addressed to the Public Inquiries and Reports Branch. A publications list is available.

87-127   NATIONAL SICKLE CELL DISEASE PROGRAM
Department of Health and Human Services
National Institutes of Health
National Heart, Lung, and Blood Institute
Federal Bldg., Rm. 504
7550 Wisconsin Ave.
Bethesda, MD 20892
(301) 496-6931

SERVICES: At the recommendation of the President, Congress appropriated funds in 1971 for a National Sickle Cell Disease Advisory Committee, which recommended the establishment of the National Sickle Cell Disease Program. Components of the program include centers to coordinate manpower, research findings, and facilities, offering a combination of research and demonstration services (fundamental research, clinical research, clinical application, treatment trials, professional and paraprofessional training and education programs, public education, consultation, screening, counseling, rehabilitation, and related activities); screening and education clinics; a mission-oriented research and development program; research project grants; public and professional education; and a hemoglobinopathy training program.

PUBLICATIONS: Consumer materials are available on sickle cell disease and health care facilities. Professional materials are available on sickle cell disease.

HIGHWAY TRAFFIC SAFETY

**87-128 NATIONAL HIGHWAY TRAFFIC SAFETY
ADMINISTRATION (NHTSA)**
Office of Consumer Affairs
Department of Transportation
400 Seventh St., SW, (NOA-40)
Washington, DC 20590
(202) 366-5965
(202) 366-0123 (Auto Safety Hotline—Metropolitan
    Washington DC)
(800) 424-9393 (Auto Safety Hotline)

SERVICES: NHTSA, established in 1966, works to reduce
highway traffic deaths and injuries by promulgating vehicle standards, providing consumer information on vehicle and highway
safety, and issuing standards for highway and traffic safety. As
part of its health promotion activities, NHTSA provides technical and training assistance to states, awards grants to highway
safety programs, and conducts research in occupant protection.
It publishes a variety of informational brochures; conducts health
promotion and risk reduction public educational programs that
promote the use of seat belts, child safety seats, and automatic
protection; and informs the public on the hazards of drunk driving. NHTSA also maintains a toll-free hotline for consumer
complaints on auto safety and child safety seats and requests for
information on recalls.
PUBLICATIONS: Consumer materials are available on safety
belts and child safety seats, drunk driving, auto safety, audiovisual materials, and auto manufacturer defect campaigns. Professional materials include curriculum guides (elementary and
secondary level), manuals, public service announcements, and
summaries of state legislation.

INDIAN HEALTH SERVICE

87-129 INDIAN HEALTH SERVICE (IHS)
Department of Health and Human Services
Health Resources and Services Administration
Parklawn Bldg., Rm. 5A-55
5600 Fishers Lane
Rockville, MD 20857
(301) 443-1083

SERVICES: The Indian Health Service provides comprehensive health services on medical, dental, and environmental health programs through IHS and tribally contracted hospitals, health centers, school health centers, and health stations. Special program concentrations are in alcoholism, suicide, accidents, maternal and child health, nutrition, and otitis media (inflammation of the middle ear).

PUBLICATIONS: Professional materials are available on Native Americans, health care services, and nutrition.

INFECTIOUS DISEASES

87-130   **ARMY MEDICAL RESEARCH INSTITUTE OF**
         INFECTIOUS DISEASES
         MEDICAL LIBRARY
         Department of the Army
         Office of the Surgeon General of the Army
         Army Medical Research and Development Command
         Bldg. 1425, SGRD UIA-L
         Fort Detrick
         Frederick, MD 21701
         (301) 663-2720

SERVICES: The library's areas of interest include medical
defense against biological warfare, high hazard infectious diseases, metabolism and infection, vaccine development and production, radiation and infection, antiviral therapy, aerobiology,
and toxins. It answers inquiries; provides reference and copying services and information on R&D in progress; distributes
publications; makes direct and interlibrary loans and referrals
to other sources of information; and permits on-site use of its
collections, subject to facility and personnel limitations.

87-131   **CENTERS FOR DISEASE CONTROL (CDC)**
         Public Affairs Office
         Department of Health and Human Services
         Bldg. 1, Rm. 2067
         1600 Clifton Rd., NE
         Atlanta, GA 30333
         (404) 329-3286
         (404) 329-3524 (Public Inquiries Office)

SERVICES: CDC has nationwide programs for the prevention and control of infectious and other preventable diseases, including malnutrition, disease control techniques and communicable diseases, foreign and interstate quarantine activities, epidemic and disaster aid, epidemiology, venereal diseases, tuberculosis, immunization, lead-based paint poisoning, upgrading performance and licensure of clinical laboratories engaged in interstate commerce, family planning, congenital defects, occupational safety and health, and health education. The Public Affairs Office deals directly with the public regarding program activities. It will direct technical inquiries for information to the proper programs within the centers or to such services as the library. Other services are available to state and local health departments and to other federal agencies.

PUBLICATIONS: *Morbidity and Mortality Weekly Report;* various *Surveillance Reports* dealing with specific diseases or categories of diseases; *Current Literature on Venereal Diseases* (annotated bibliography); *Tuberculosis* (irregular publications on incidence and distribution); *Immunization* (covering production and distribution of biologics); training materials for public health practitioners; materials on reproductive health and health education; and *Registry of Toxic Effects of Chemical Substances.* Subscription information on the *Morbidity and Mortality Weekly Report* and information on other CDC publications are available from the Public Inquiries Office.

87-132 NATIONAL INSTITUTE OF ALLERGY AND INFECTIOUS DISEASES (NIAID)
Office of Communications
Department of Health and Human Services
Bldg. 31, Rm. 7A-32
9000 Rockville Pike
Bethesda, MD 20892
(301) 496-5717

SERVICES: NIAID conducts and supports research on infectious and allergic diseases and on immunology. The institute is seeking to learn more about the process of bacterial and viral infections and continues to work on the development of antiviral substances. It has major responsibility for research on the immune system. NIAID is organized into program areas that pertain to grants and contracts awarded to scientists in universities and private research institutions. Technical innovations that are being pursued include recombinant DNA technology and hybridoma cell fusion.

PUBLICATIONS: Consumer materials are available on allergies, bacterial meningitis, sinusitis, poison ivy allergy, mold allergy, pollen allergy, dust allergy, insect allergy, asthma, rabies, viruses, sexually transmitted diseases, viral hepatitis, genital herpes, Reye's syndrome, toxoplasmosis, tuberculosis, and the immune system. Professional materials are available on research reagents, tissue typing antisera, cholera, asthma, recombinant DNA research, immunology, sexually transmitted diseases, and virology. Selected reports are available from the National Technical Information Service, Springfield, VA 22161. A publications list is available.

INTERNATIONAL HEALTH

87-133 FOGARTY INTERNATIONAL CENTER
Department of Health and Human Services
National Institutes of Health (NIH)
Bldg. 38A, Rm. 604
9000 Rockville Pike
Bethesda, MD 20892
(301) 496-4627

SERVICES: The center, a division of NIH, furthers international collaboration in biomedical and behavioral sciences; examines major international biomedical research issues through a program of advanced studies; supports scholars in residence, international conferences, and postdoctoral research and exchange of scientists between the United States and other countries; coordinates NIH biomedical and behavioral research at the international level; and acts as liaison in international affairs between NIH and other governmental and international agencies. Its primary areas of interest are aspects of biomedical and behavioral sciences having international implications. Available publications are distributed in response to requests. Telephone inquiries are referred to appropriate offices.

PUBLICATIONS: Conference proceedings and comparative health studies (especially China and the USSR); *Annual Report on NIH International Activities*. A publications list is available.

87-134 OFFICE OF INTERNATIONAL HEALTH (OIH)
Department of Health and Human Services
Parklawn Bldg., Rm. 18-87
5600 Fishers Lane
Rockville, MD 20857
(301) 443-1774

SERVICES: OIH provides support to the Assistant Secretary for Health in developing policy and coordinates activities of the Public Health Service agencies of DHHS in the field of international health.   It works closely with the World Health Organization and other international organizations.   OIH oversees PHS participation in more than 25 binational health agreements. Several desk officers serve as experts on various regions of the world.   OIH will respond to questions regarding U.S. participation in international health agreements and programs.

PUBLICATIONS: OIH does not distribute publications, but its publications may be purchased from the National Technical Information Service, Springfield, VA 22161. Professional materials are available on health planning, health manpower, breastfeeding, communicable diseases, and international health.   A publications list is available.

MEDICAL BIOENGINEERING

87-135 ARMY BIOMEDICAL RESEARCH AND DEVELOPMENT LABORATORY
Library
Department of the Army
Office of the Surgeon General of the Army
Army Medical Research and Development Command
Bldg. 568
Fort Detrick
Frederick, MD 21701-5010
(301) 663-2502

SERVICES: The laboratory (formerly known as the Army Medical Bioengineering Research and Development Laboratory) conducts engineering research and development of military medical equipment on a continuing basis for the Army and on an "as required" basis for the Navy and Air Force. It is responsible for the construction of initial pilot prototypes and test models and for the production of limited quantities of medical materials to support urgent military requirements. It conducts the Surgeon General's research and development program in integrated pest management systems, including materials, methods, equipment, and concepts, as well as environmental health engineering research in support of the Surgeon General's responsibilities in air and water pollution control and solid waste and pesticides disposal, including management of the intramural and extramural portions of the Army Medical Research and Development Command's Environmental Quality Protection Program. The library answers inquiries and provides reference and interlibrary loan services and reprints of laboratory staff publications. Services are primarily for the laboratory's research staff, but outside requests are filled as time permits.

MENTAL HEALTH

87-136 EMERGENCY SERVICES BRANCH
Department of Health and Human Services
Alcohol, Drug Abuse, and Mental Health Administration
National Institute of Mental Health
Parklawn Bldg., Rm. 7C-02
5600 Fishers Lane
Rockville, MD 20857
(301) 443-4735

SERVICES: The Emergency Services Branch (formerly the
Center for Mental Health Studies of Emergencies) performs the
following functions: coordinates National Institute of Mental
Health activities relating to the mental health needs of persons
in emergency conditions arising from crises in the physical environment; analyzes and evaluates current research and development; stimulates, develops, and supports research and training programs; collaborates with the Public Health Service, the
Federal Emergency Management Agency, and other public and
private agencies to administer crisis counseling programs in areas that have been declared disaster areas by the President of
the United States; and develops and disseminates relevant educational materials. Services of the center are for use by mental
health professionals and state and local agencies involved with
emergency planning.
PUBLICATIONS: A publications list is available.

**87-137 NATIONAL INSTITUTE OF MENTAL HEALTH (NIMH)
DIVISION OF BIOMETRY AND APPLIED SCIENCES**
Department of Health and Human Services
Alcohol, Drug Abuse, and Mental Health Administration

Parklawn Bldg., Rm. 18C-07
5600 Fishers Lane
Rockville, MD 20857
(301) 443-3343

SERVICES: The principal areas of interest of the Division of Biometry and Applied Sciences, formerly the Division of Biometry and Epidemiology, are information on epidemiology of mental disorders, health services research in mental health, provision of mental health care in primary health care settings, and economics of mental health; information on patients in public and private mental hospitals, community mental health centers, psychiatric services in general hospitals, outpatient facilities, and transitional facilities; and reports on trends, use of facilities, socioeconomic data, classification of mental disorders, application of mental health statistics, and other related special studies, including mathematical statistics concerned with experimental design and methods of statistical analysis. The division's current publications and reprints are available to interested persons and are used to answer queries from the public.

HOLDINGS: More than 500 publications and reprints, based on reports from some 2,500 mental health facilities.

PUBLICATIONS: Special reports on the diverse subjects listed under services above. Statistical data are routinely published in one of two forms: the *Mental Health Statistical Note Series* or the *Mental Health Service System Reports* (Series: *AN-Epidemiology; BN-Needs Assessment and Evaluation; CN-National Statistics; DN-Health/Mental Health Research; EN-Mental Health Economics; FN-Information Systems; GN-Methodology*), formerly the *Series Reports on Mental Health Statistics* (Series A through D). The *Mental Health Statistical Note Series* presents brief summaries of data focusing on a limited topic or a specific question. The *Mental Health Service System Reports* series presents detailed data on broader subject matters, including descriptive data on mental health facilities, patients served, staffing, analytical and special studies, methodological advances, new analytical techniques, and special conference and committee reports. The reserialized reports are targeted more appropriately to specific audiences and include a mix of new publications and reissues of selected reports from the old series, which are of continuing interest and relevance. A publications list is available.

**87-138   NATIONAL INSTITUTE OF MENTAL HEALTH (NIMH)
SCIENTIFIC INFORMATION BRANCH**
Public Inquiries Section
Department of Health and Human Services
Alcohol, Drug Abuse, and Mental Health Administration
Parklawn Bldg., Rm. 15C-05
5600 Fishers Lane
Rockville, MD 20857
(301) 443-4513

SERVICES: The Scientific Information Branch of NIMH has the following specific functions: collecting scientific, technical, and other information on mental illness and health from the staff and operating components of NIMH and other outside sources; classifying, storing, and retrieving information; and preparing special publications for professional and lay audiences.   The Public Inquiries Section answers general inquiries from the public and provides information on mental health exhibits and films. General inquiries are answered within two weeks, but publication requests may take longer.
DATABASE: NIMH prepared the MENTAL HEALTH ABSTRACTS DATABASE during the years 1969 through 1982. Beginning in 1983, updates to the database are prepared by IFI/Plenum Data Company in Wilmington, Delaware.   The database is accessible to the public through DIALOG.
PUBLICATIONS: Materials are available on behavioral problems, learning disorders, developmental problems, childhood hyperactivity, mental health administration, schizophrenia, depressive illness, and psychological stress. A publications list is available.

**87-139   PRESIDENT'S COMMITTEE ON MENTAL RETARDATION
(PCMR)**

Department of Health and Human Services
North Bldg., Rm. 4723
330 Independence Ave., SW
Washington, DC 20201
(202) 245-7634

SERVICES: The committee advises the President on appropriate ways to provide for mentally retarded citizens and how to prevent this type of disability. Areas of concern are full citizenship, prevention of biomedical and environmental causes of retardation, community support services, international activities, and public information. PCMR sponsors forums and conferences and prepares an annual report to the President. The committee serves as a liaison between the federal sector and state and local agencies.

PUBLICATIONS: Materials are available on the legal rights of the mentally retarded, employment, service programs, and mental retardation. A publications list is available.

MILITARY MEDICINE ADMINISTRATION

**87-140   DIRECTORATE OF HEALTH CARE SUPPORT
BIOMETRICS DIVISION**
Department of the Air Force
Office of the Surgeon General of the Air Force
Headquarters USAF
AFOMS/SGSB
San Antonio, TX 78235-5000
(512) 536-3983

Located at: Bldg. 150, Rm. 102
            Brooks Air Force Base, TX 78235-5000

SERVICES: The Biometrics Division provides approved researchers with data on Air Force Medical Treatment Facility
(MTF) analyses, frequency, or prevalency of specific illnesses;
diagnostic data from medical records; and information on the
methodology of collecting, recording, and analyzing medical
records and implementing data codes for computerized operations.   Data from all admission (inpatient) records have been
taken from clinical charts and stored on computer media. Statistical tabulations, monthly hospital analyses, and diagnostic
listings are maintained for each Air Force MTF.

**87-141   HEALTH SERVICES COMMAND
PUBLIC AFFAIRS OFFICE**
Department of the Army
Fort Sam Houston
San Antonio, TX 78234-6000
(512) 221-6213

SERVICES: The areas of interest of the Public Affairs Office include military health services, medical facilities, medical units, and medical professional training; military preventive medicine; and Army health standards. The office answers inquiries, provides advisory and reference services, and makes referrals.

PUBLICATIONS: *Mercury* (monthly newspaper); *Health of the Army* (quarterly); and professional medical audiovisual productions.

87-142 OFFICE OF THE SURGEON GENERAL OF THE AIR FORCE
Congressional and Public Affairs Branch
Department of the Air Force
Bldg. 5681
Bolling Air Force Base
Washington, DC 20332
(202) 767-5046

SERVICES: The Office of the Surgeon General of the Air Force develops and administers medical benefits programs for Air Force personnel and eligible dependents and civilians. Inquiries concerning eligibility may be directed to this office. In addition, the Office of the Surgeon General has implemented a Consumer Health Education Program, which provides guidance and material on disease prevention and health promotion to beneficiaries.

87-143 OFFICE OF THE SURGEON GENERAL OF THE ARMY
Department of the Army
5111 Leesburg Pike, Rm. 635
Falls Church, VA 22041-3258
(703) 756-0000

SERVICES: The Office of the Surgeon General of the Army is responsible for worldwide U.S. Army health plans and policies; personnel management of health professionals, including graduate health education; Army health standards; and military medical research and development. The office answers Army health care inquiries. Other inquiries are answered subject to material and personnel limitations. Advisory and reference services are limited according to time and effort required. Costs for information retrieval are based on actual computer time and man-hours expended.

HOLDINGS: Information holdings include a client-oriented drug abuse reporting system, a Medical R&D Scientific and Technical Information Activity, and a Patient Administration and Biostatistics Activity.

PUBLICATIONS: Department of the Army pamphlets (40 series); *Department of the Army Regulations* (40 series).

87-144   OFFICE OF THE SURGEON GENERAL OF THE ARMY
PATIENT ADMINISTRATION DIVISION
Department of the Army
5111 Leesburg Pike, Rm. 611
Falls Church, VA 22041-3258
(703) 756-0102

SERVICES: Medical benefits programs for Army personnel and eligible civilians, including dependents, are developed and administered by this office; it also responds to inquiries about eligibility for benefits.

87-145   OFFICE OF THE SURGEONS GENERAL OF THE ARMY
AND AIR FORCE
JOINT MEDICAL LIBRARY
The Pentagon, Rm. 1B-473
Washington, DC 20310-2300
(202) 695-5752

SERVICES: The main areas of interest of the Joint Medical Library are medical specialties, medical personnel, medical and hospital administration, nursing, public health, and military medical history. The library answers inquiries, provides reference services, and makes referrals and interlibrary loans.

HOLDINGS: The library's holdings consist of approximately 12,000 books and 430 journal subscriptions, files of military medical publications, annual reports of the Surgeons General, and medical school catalogs.

NATIONAL HEALTH SERVICE CORPS

87-146   NATIONAL HEALTH SERVICE CORPS (NHSC)
Department of Health and Human Services
Health Resources and Services Administration
Parklawn Bldg., Rm. 7A-39
5600 Fishers Lane
Rockville, MD 20857
(301) 443-2900

SERVICES: NHSC, in cooperation with regional offices, de-
termines which health manpower shortage areas may have physicians, dentists, and other health personnel assigned to complete a
period of service in repayment for educational scholarships. The
corps then monitors the performance of these personnel, evaluates the results of placements, and promotes the development of
permanent health care delivery systems by encouraging the as-
signees, after completing their period of service with the corps,
to remain and continue to serve in the selected areas. NHSC
answers inquiries, makes referrals, and provides pamphlets and
brochures.

**87-147   NATIONAL HEALTH SERVICE CORPS (NHSC)
DIVISION OF HEALTH SERVICES SCHOLARSHIPS**
Department of Health and Human Services
Health Resources and Services Administration
Parklawn Bldg., Room 7-16
5600 Fishers Lane
Rockville, MD 20857
(301) 443-1650

SERVICES: NHSC's Division of Health Services Scholarships provides scholarships and loans to students in the health professions in exchange for a commitment to work in an underserved area upon graduation. Different scholarship arrangements are associated with various lengths of service. Health professionals are sent to communities with one primary care physician (or fewer) per 3,500 people. Information about NHSC's scholarship program only—the possibility of obtaining financial assistance—is available from this office.

NATIONAL INSTITUTES OF HEALTH PROGRAMS

**87-148   NATIONAL INSTITUTES OF HEALTH (NIH)
DIVISION OF PUBLIC INFORMATION**
Department of Health and Human Services
Bldg. 1, Rm. 307
9000 Rockville Pike
Bethesda, MD 20892
(301) 496-5787

SERVICES: The Division of Public Information is responsible for developing and disseminating materials relating to NIH as a whole and for providing support services to the various institutes and other organizations that comprise NIH. In responding to public inquiries, the division will refer requests to the most appropriate institute. The division consists of the Editorial Operations Branch, the News Branch, and the Audiovisual Branch. The Editorial Operations Branch reviews and edits materials produced by the various components of NIH and edits speeches and other presentations made by upper-level NIH personnel. The News Branch develops press releases, assists in the production of articles relating to medical issues, and reviews articles produced outside of NIH for content. The Audiovisual Branch produces a regular monthly series of health issues interviews with scientists for use on the radio, produces public service announcements for radio and television, assists NIH components in the development of films and exhibits, and approves all such films and exhibits. Materials produced by the various NIH institutes, as listed in the *NIH Publications List,* should be requested from the appropriate institute.

DATABASE: In November 1986, NIH announced the availability of the HUMAN NUTRITION RESEARCH AND INFORMATION MANAGEMENT (HNRIM) interagency database, which provides information on human nutrition research and research training activities supported in whole or in part by the Federal Government. Each participating agency (at present, the Department of Health and Human Services, Department of Agriculture, Veterans Administration, Agency for International Development, Department of Defense, and National Marine Fisheries Service of the Department of Commerce) assembles and submits its own data to NIH. Data from the participating agencies are combined into a central HNRIM database and are updated quarterly. The database contains approximately 4,000 nutrition and training projects and can be purchased from the National Technical Information Service, Springfield, VA 22161.

PUBLICATIONS: *NIH Almanac* (annual); *NIH Publications List* (annual).

**87-149 NATIONAL INSTITUTES OF HEALTH (NIH)
DIVISION OF RESEARCH SERVICES**
Department of Health and Human Services
Bldg. 12A, Rm. 4007
9000 Rockville Pike
Bethesda, MD 20892
(301) 496-5795

SERVICES: The Division of Research Services, established in 1966, provides support services for scientists conducting research in NIH laboratories. The division is organized to provide services and products at each of four sequential steps in every biomedical research project: planning, making available models and substrates, manipulating and measuring research materials, and recording and communicating research results. The division includes the Library Branch, which possesses or has access to virtually all published biomedical knowledge; the Veterinary Resources Branch, which provides animal models and proper facilities for their use; the Biomedical Engineering and Instrumentation Branch, which assists in planning the use of research materials and measurement of results; and the Medical Arts and Photography Branch, which assists in the communication of research results to the scientific community. Its library, located in Building 10, Room IL25B, at the above address, which includes approximately 90,000 monographs and 200,000 bound volumes of journals, is open to the public. The library's online search capability is available only to NIH employees.

PUBLICATION: *Annual Report.*

NAVAL MEDICAL RESEARCH

87-150 NAVAL HEALTH RESEARCH CENTER (NHRC)
WILKINS BIOMEDICAL LIBRARY
Department of the Navy
Naval Medical Research and Development Command
Cabrillo Memorial Dr., Bldg. 306
P.O. Box 85122
San Diego, CA 92138
(619) 225-6640

SERVICES: The library's areas of interest are naval medicine, stress medicine, epidemiology, environmental physiology, environmental and social medicine, biological sciences, sleep research, and work physiology. In addition to books, journals, and reports, the library maintains a collection of Audio-Digest medical tapes in internal medicine, psychiatry, and emergency medicine. The library answers inquiries; provides advisory, reference, literature-searching, and current-awareness services; and makes direct and interlibrary loans and referrals to other sources of information. Services are primarily for NHRC employees, but the public may use the facilities on a time-available basis.

87-151 NAVAL MEDICAL RESEARCH INSTITUTE (NMRI)
Department of the Navy
Naval Medical Research and Development Command
Rockville Pike, Bldg. 17
Bethesda, MD 20814-5055
(202) 295-2186

SERVICES: The Naval Medical Research Institute conducts life sciences research directly related to Naval and Marine Corps requirements. Its major areas of interest are military medicine, medical research, pathology, surgery, hyperbaric medicine, microbiology, biochemistry, bioengineering, transplantation, and stress psychology. The institute's library serves primarily the Department of Defense and other federal agencies. Subject to availability of material and personnel, it will provide limited referral and interlibrary loan services to others.

PUBLICATIONS: The institute's reports of research are available from the National Technical Information Service, Springfield, VA 22161.

**87-152   NAVAL SUBMARINE MEDICAL RESEARCH
                LABORATORY**
Department of the Navy
Naval Medical Research and Development Command
Naval Submarine Base New London
P.O. Box 900
Groton, CT 06349-5900
(203) 449-3263

SERVICES: The laboratory's areas of interest are psychophysiology of audition and vision, human factors engineering, physiology of submarine atmosphere, respiratory physiology, diving research, decompression studies, personnel research (selection, motivation, performance, effects of stress), cold weather medicine, and human aspects of military operations. It answers inquiries and makes limited interlibrary loans.

PUBLICATIONS: The laboratory produces technical and special reports.

**87-153   OFFICE OF NAVAL RESEARCH
                LIBRARY**
Department of the Navy
Ballston Tower No. 1, Rm. 633
800 N. Quincy St.

Arlington, VA 22217-5000
(202) 696-4415

SERVICES: The library's primary areas of interest are current research and development in the fields of physical, biological, medical, social, and Naval sciences.   The library answers inquiries and makes interlibrary loans and referrals to other sources of information.   Services are limited according to the time and effort required.

NEUROLOGICAL AND COMMUNICATIVE DISORDERS

**87-154   NATIONAL INSTITUTE OF NEUROLOGICAL AND
COMMUNICATIVE DISORDERS
AND STROKE (NINCDS)**
Office of Scientific and Health Reports
Department of Health and Human Services
National Institutes of Health
Bldg. 31, Rm. 8A-06
9000 Rockville Pike
Bethesda, MD 20892
(301) 496-5924

SERVICES: NINCDS, established in 1950 as the National
Institute of Neurological Diseases and Blindness, became the
National Institute of Neurological Diseases and Communicative
Disorders and Stroke in 1975. NINCDS conducts and supports
research and research training on the causes, prevention, diagnosis, and treatment of neurological and communicative disorders and stroke. It awards grants for research projects, program
projects, and center grants; provides training support to institutions and fellowships to individuals in the field of neurological
and communicative disorders and stroke; conducts intramural
and collaborative research; and collects and disseminates research information.

PUBLICATIONS: Consumer materials are available on acous-
tic neuroma, amyotrophic lateral sclerosis, aphasia, autism, cere-
bral palsy, dementias, epilepsy, Friedreich's ataxia, Huntington's
disease, multiple sclerosis, muscular dystrophy, myasthenia
gravis, neurofibromatosis, Parkinson's disease, shingles, spina
bifida, spinal cord injury, stuttering, torsion dystonia, stroke,
head injury, Gaucher's disease, Niemann-Pick disease, Fabry's

disease, Tay-Sachs disease, Farber's disease, metachromatic leukodystrophy, and lipid storage diseases. Professional materials are available on neurological disorders, stroke, epilepsy, communicative disorders, Alzheimer's disease, research and training programs, speech disorders, and spinal cord injuries. A publications list is available.

NUCLEAR SAFETY

87-155 NUCLEAR SAFETY INFORMATION CENTER
Oak Ridge National Laboratory
Bldg. 9201-3 (MS-5)
P.O. Box Y
Oak Ridge, TN 37831
(615) 574-0391

SERVICES: Sponsored by the Nuclear Regulatory Commission, the center serves the nuclear community by collecting, storing, evaluating, and disseminating nuclear safety information generated throughout the world. The center's scope of interest is on information generated by operating nuclear facilities, principally nuclear power plants. It answers technical inquiries, prepares special bibliographies, provides technical consulting services, and permits on-site use of its document collection. Services are provided free to sponsoring agencies and their contractors and on a cost-recovery basis to others.

PUBLICATIONS: The technical progress review *Nuclear Safety* (bimonthly, sponsored by the Department of Energy and the Nuclear Regulatory Commission); state-of-the-art reports; and topical bibliographies.

OCCUPATIONAL SAFETY AND HEALTH

87-156 CLEARINGHOUSE FOR OCCUPATIONAL SAFETY AND HEALTH INFORMATION
Department of Health and Human Services
Centers for Disease Control
National Institute for Occupational Safety and Health (NIOSH)
4676 Columbia Pkwy.
Cincinnati, OH 45226
(513) 533-8385

SERVICES: The clearinghouse, established in 1976, provides technical information support for NIOSH research programs and provides information to others on request. Services include reference and referral, interlibrary loans, and information about NIOSH studies. Its library consists of approximately 12,000 books and 1,100 periodicals in two library locations, with no restrictions on their on-site use.

DATABASE: The online NIOSH database, NIOSHTIC, indexes current and retrospective materials dating back to the 1800s, covering the field of occupational safety and health. Sources indexed by this database include journal articles, materials from the International Labor Organization's Clearinghouse for Occupational Safety and Health, the International Occupational Safety and Health Information Center database, and references from *NIOSH Criteria Documents* and *Current Intelligence Bulletins.* The database is available through DIALOG.

PUBLICATIONS: Professional materials are available on occupational health, hazardous substances, and safety.

87-157 NATIONAL INSTITUTE FOR OCCUPATIONAL SAFETY AND HEALTH (NIOSH)

OFFICE OF INFORMATION
Department of Health and Human Services
Centers for Disease Control
Bldg. 1, Rm. 3041
1600 Clifton Rd., NE
Atlanta, GA 30333
(404) 329-3345

SERVICES: Serving as the point of contact for inquiries relating to the policies of NIOSH, the Office of Information answers questions of a nontechnical nature in the occupational safety and health field and provides single copies of NIOSH publications to visitors. Telephone or mail requests for publications and inquiries of a technical nature are referred to the Clearinghouse for Occupational Safety and Health Information (87-156).

DATABASE: The REGISTRY OF TOXIC EFFECTS OF CHEMICAL SUBSTANCES (RTECS), is an online, interactive version of the NIOSH publication *Registry of Toxic Effects of Chemical Substances,* formerly called the *Toxic Substances List.* Maintained by NIOSH and compiled annually, it contains basic acute and chronic toxicity data for more than 78,000 potentially toxic chemicals. Records include toxicity data, chemical identifiers, exposure standards, and status under various federal regulations and programs. The file can be searched by chemical identifiers, type of effect, or other criteria through MEDLARS (87-055).

**87-158   OCCUPATIONAL SAFETY AND HEALTH
          ADMINISTRATION (OSHA)**
Office of Information and Consumer Affairs
Department of Labor
200 Constitution Ave., NW, Rm. N-3637
Washington, DC 20210
(202) 523-8148

SERVICES: Under the Occupational Safety and Health Act of 1970, OSHA was created to encourage employers and employees to reduce workplace hazards and to implement new or improved safety and health programs; to establish separate but dependent responsibilities and rights for employers and employees to achieve better safety and health conditions; to maintain a reporting and record-keeping system to monitor job-related injuries and illnesses; to develop mandatory job safety and health standards and to enforce them; and to provide for the development, analysis, evaluation, and approval of state occupational safety and health programs. The act also provides six distinct provisions for protecting the safety and health of federal workers on the job. OSHA encourages a broad range of voluntary workplace improvement efforts, including consultation programs, training and education efforts, grants to increase safety and health compliance, and a variety of other similar programs.

PUBLICATIONS: Materials are available on occupational health, occupational safety, asbestos, back injuries, federal regulations, hearing, accidents, statistical data, and carcinogens. Some materials are available from the National Technical Information Service, Springfield, VA 22161 or the Superintendent of Documents, U.S. Government Printing Office, Washington, DC 20402. A print and audiovisual publications list is available on request, with a self-addressed mailing label.

ORPHAN DRUGS AND RARE DISEASES

87-159 NATIONAL INFORMATION CENTER ON ORPHAN DRUGS AND RARE DISEASES (NICODARD)
P.O. Box 1133
Washington, DC 20013-1133
(202) 429-9091 (Virginia and Metropolitan Washington, DC)
(800) 336-4797

SERVICES: NICODARD, a component of the ODPHP Health Information Center (87-118), was established in October 1984. Using the ODPHP referral process, the NICODARD staff answer inquiries on rare diseases (defined as those with a prevalence in the United States of 200,000 or fewer cases) and on orphan drugs (medicines not widely researched or available). Requesters may call or write NICODARD directly. The center is a service of the Office of Disease Prevention and Health Promotion, DHHS, and is sponsored by the Orphan Products Board, Food and Drug Administration, DHHS.

PUBLICATIONS: Materials under preparation include rare disease profiles, fact sheets, and a directory of educational materials.

PATHOLOGY

87-160 ARMED FORCES INSTITUTE OF PATHOLOGY (AFIP)
Department of Defense
14th St. and Alaska Ave., NW
Washington, DC 20306-6000
(202) 576-2934

SERVICES: Under a Department of Defense charter, AFIP is a joint agency of the Army, Navy, and Air Force. It is under the management control of the Surgeon General of the Army. AFIP's areas of interest cover all aspects of pathology, including subspecialties such as neuropathology and ophthalmic, forensic, oral, veterinary, geographic, environmental, and radiologic pathology. Information resources consist of the AFIP Repository (tissues, slides, case records, etc.), which includes 29 registries, each dealing with one field of pathology; a library collection of approximately 17,500 books, 325 periodical titles, and 2,000 reports; and a Medical Museum divided into four main areas: the Hammond Hall of Pathology, the Brinton Hall of History, the Silliphant Hall of Current Events, and the Billings Hall of Instruments, which contains the world's largest microscope collection. The institute answers inquiries and provides a worldwide consulting service that, on an emergency basis, can be completed in 24 hours; provides numerous postgraduate courses in advanced pathology; makes referrals; lends pathologic, photographic, and other educational materials to federal medical services, museums, medical schools, scientific institutions, and qualified professionals; conducts experimental, statistical, and morphological research; and permits on-site use of its collections. Services are primarily for medical, dental, and veterinary pathologists and related professionals. Facilities include the 16-room Center for Advanced Study in Pathology (CASP) for professional use. The

Medical Museum is open daily from 10:00 a.m. to 5:00 p.m., Monday through Friday, and from 12 noon to 5:00 p.m., Saturday and Sunday; it is closed on Thanksgiving Day, Christmas Eve, Christmas, New Year's Eve, and New Year's Day.

PUBLICATIONS: *Atlas of Tumor Pathology* (39 individual pathology fascicles, now in 2nd series); a newsletter, journal articles, books, syllabi, reports, and pamphlets. Approximately 200 professional papers are published annually. A publications list is available.

PHARMACEUTICALS

87-161 CENTER FOR DRUGS AND BIOLOGICS
MEDICAL LIBRARY
Department of Health and Human Services
Food and Drug Administration
Parklawn Bldg., Rm. 11B-07
5600 Fishers Lane
Rockville, MD 20857
(301) 443-1538

SERVICES: The library's principal areas of interest are pharmacology, toxicology, drug therapy and adverse reactions, biologics, biotechnology, epidemiology, immunology, clinical medicine, chemistry, pharmacy, food and drug law, biostatistics, veterinary medicine, and management. It answers inquiries, provides reference and literature-searching services, makes interlibrary loans on a cooperative basis, and permits on-site use of its collection. Reference services to non-FDA personnel are limited.

87-162 CENTER FOR DRUGS AND BIOLOGICS
LEGISLATIVE, PROFESSIONAL, AND CONSUMER
AFFAIRS BRANCH
Department of Health and Human Services
Food and Drug Administration
Office of Compliance
Division of Regulatory Affairs
Parklawn Bldg.
5600 Fishers Lane (HFN-365)
Rockville, MD 20857

(301) 295-8012 (Inquiries)
(301) 443-3170 (Publications)
(301) 295-8012 (Drug Approvals)

SERVICES: The Legislative, Professional, and Consumer Affairs Branch of the Center for Drugs and Biologics, formerly called the Bureau of Drugs, responds to inquiries covering the entire spectrum of drug issues and develops center and agency responses to drug information requests under the Freedom of Information Act (FOI). Inquiries are received by telephone and mail; however, all FOI requests should be in writing, addressed to FOI Staff (HFW-35), 5600 Fishers Lane, Rockville, MD 20857. For product approvals, obtain information by telephone only from the drug approvals number listed above.

PUBLICATIONS: Professional materials are available on pharmaceuticals, poison control centers, federal regulations, and drug approvals.

87-163   FDA FIELD FACILITIES
Office of Regional Operations
Department of Health and Human Services
Food and Drug Administration
Parklawn Bldg., Rm. 13-61
5600 Fishers Lane (HFC 100)
Rockville, MD 20857
(301) 443-6230

SERVICES: FDA field activities are primarily concerned with the chemical, biological (microbiology and entomology), physical, and sensory analysis of foods, drugs, medical devices, and cosmetics for the purpose of enforcing the Food, Drug, and Cosmetic Act and related laws. All laboratories listed below answer questions pertaining to analytical methodology. Although the functions of the laboratories are similar, some specialize in specific areas. The Chicago laboratory specializes in computer-assisted analysis; the Denver laboratory, in tissue residue analysis; the Kansas City laboratory, in total diet studies (analysis of pesticides, heavy metals, etc.); the New Orleans laboratory, in mycotoxin analysis; and the Atlanta laboratory, in nutritional analysis.

PUBLICATIONS: Analytical methodologies developed by FDA scientists are published in the open literature. Most of the methods are published in the *Journal of the Association of Official Analytical Chemists (JAOAC)* and in the *Official Methods of Analysis of the AOAC;* however, FDA also publishes analytical manuals covering specific subject areas. Most of these manuals can be obtained by writing to the Executive Director of Regional Operations, Division of Field Science / HFO-600, Food and Drug Administration, 5600 Fishers Lane, Rockville, MD 20857. The manuals include the *Drug Autoanalysis Manual; Food Additives Analytical Manual; Microanalytical Manual; Pesticide Analytical Manual,* 2 vols.; and *Bacteriological Analytical Manual* (all available from the Superintendent of Documents, U.S. Government Printing Office, Washington, D.C. 20402).

FDA DISTRICT LABORATORIES

Atlanta District
Food and Drug Administration Laboratory
60 8th St., NE
Atlanta, GA 30309
(404) 881-7527

Baltimore District
Food and Drug Administration Laboratory
900 Madison Ave.
Baltimore, MD 21201
(301) 962-3790

Boston District
Food and Drug Administration Laboratory
585 Commercial St.
Boston, MA 02109
(617) 223-5699

Brooklyn District
Food and Drug Administration Laboratory
850 3rd Ave.
Brooklyn, NY 11232
(212) 965-5033

Buffalo District
Food and Drug Administration Laboratory
599 Delaware Ave.
Buffalo, NY 14202
(716) 846-4494

Chicago District
Food and Drug Administration Laboratory
10 W. 35th St.
Chicago, IL 60616
(312) 353-9764

Cincinnati District
Food and Drug Administration Laboratory
1141 Central Pkwy.
Cincinnati, OH 45202
(513) 684-3512

Dallas District
Food and Drug Administration Laboratory
3032 Bryan St.
Dallas, TX 75204
(214) 767-0309

Denver District
Food and Drug Administration Laboratory
U.S. Custom House, Rm. 500
721 19th St.
Denver, CO 80202
(303) 844-4915

Detroit District
Food and Drug Administration Laboratory
1560 E. Jefferson Ave.
Detroit, MI 48207
(313) 226-7658

Kansas City District
Food and Drug Administration Laboratory
1009 Cherry St.
Kansas City, MO 64106
(816) 374-5524

Los Angeles District
Food and Drug Administration Laboratory
1521 W. Pico Blvd.
Los Angeles, CA 90015
(213) 688-3786

Minneapolis District
Food and Drug Administration Laboratory
240 Hennepin Ave.
Minneapolis, MN 55401
(612) 349-3931

New Orleans District
Food and Drug Administration Laboratory
4298 Elysian Fields Ave.
New Orleans, LA 70122
(504) 589-2471

Philadelphia District
Food and Drug Administration Laboratory
2nd and Chestnut Sts., Rm. 900
Philadelphia, PA 19106
(215) 597-4375

San Francisco District
Food and Drug Administration Laboratory
U.N. Plaza Federal Office Bldg., Rm. 526
San Francisco, CA 94102
(415) 556-4763

San Juan District
Food and Drug Administration Laboratory
P.O. Box S-4427, Old San Juan Sta.
San Juan, PR 00905
(809) 753-4443

Seattle District
Food and Drug Administration Laboratory
909 1st Ave., Rm. 5009
Seattle, WA 98174
(206) 442-5302

OTHER FDA FIELD FACILITIES

Minneapolis Center for Microbiological Investigations
Food and Drug Administration
240 Hennepin Ave.
Minneapolis, MN 55401
(612) 349-3937

National Center for Drug Analysis
Food and Drug Administration
1114 Market St., Rm. 1002
St. Louis, MO 63101
(314) 425-4135

National Center for Toxicological Research
Food and Drug Administration
Jefferson, AR 72079
(501) 541-4000

Winchester Engineering and Analytical Center
Food and Drug Administration
109 Holton St.
Winchester, MA 01890
(617) 729-5700

New York Import District
Food and Drug Administration
830 3rd Ave.
Brooklyn, NY 11232
(212) 965-5231

87-164 **OFFICE OF THE ASSOCIATE COMMISSIONER FOR**
LEGISLATION AND INFORMATION
PRESS RELATIONS STAFF
Department of Health and Human Services
Food and Drug Administration
Parklawn Bldg., Rm. 15B-42
5600 Fishers Lane
Rockville, MD 20857
(301) 443-3285

SERVICES: The Press Relations Staff answers inquiries and provides other services for the media on federal regulations concerning safety; packaging; efficacy; manufacture; labeling; toxicity; adverse or side effects; and contaminants of food, human and veterinary drugs, cosmetics, biological products, medical devices, diagnostic products, and ionizing and nonionizing radiation-emitting products and substances. The staff maintains an in-house computerized electronic bulletin board that provides access to up-to-date information on recalls, press releases, *FDA Consumer* indexes, medical device approval lists, drug approval lists, *Federal Register* summaries, and import detention summaries.

PUBLICATIONS: *FDA Consumer* (monthly magazine); enforcement reports (recalls), press releases, informational and educational materials, fact sheets, reprints, and speeches. A publications list is available.

PHYSICAL FITNESS

**87-165   PRESIDENT'S COUNCIL ON PHYSICAL FITNESS AND
           SPORTS (PCPFS)**
Department of Health and Human Services
405 5th St., NW, Suite 7103
Washington, DC 20001
(202) 272-3430

SERVICES: PCPFS is an outgrowth of the President's Council on Youth Fitness, which was established in 1956. It conducts a public service advertising program, prepares educational materials, and cooperates with governmental and private groups to promote the development of physical fitness leadership, facilities, and programs. PCPFS also works with schools, clubs, recreation agencies, and major employers on program design and implementation; advises federal agencies on the conduct of fitness-related programs; and offers a variety of testing, recognition, and incentive programs for individuals, institutions, and organizations.

PUBLICATIONS: Materials are available on exercise, school physical education programs, corporate fitness, physical fitness for youth and adults, jogging, walking, aquadynamics, weight training, and sports medicine. *President's Council on Physical Fitness and Sports Newsletter* (bimonthly); *Physical Fitness/Sports Medicine* (quarterly bibliography). A publications list is available.

POISONS AND ANTIDOTES

**87-166 CENTER FOR DRUGS AND BIOLOGICS
POISON CONTROL BRANCH**
Department of Health and Human Services
Food and Drug Administration
5600 Fishers Lane
Rockville, MD 20857

SERVICES: The mission of the Poison Control Branch was to evaluate potential acute toxic hazards of drugs, other household chemicals, and plants. The branch maintained a collection of millions of poison reports, data on antidotes (if any), and ingredients of new products, supplied by manufacturers of drugs and household products. It provided 600 affiliated poison control centers with information regarding antidotes and ingredients of products. With the disbanding of the Poison Control Branch late in 1986, the American Association of Poison Control Centers has assumed the national leadership role for poison control centers in the United States and has established certification criteria for regional poison control centers. The centers have a wide variety of toxicology resources, including a computerized database covering 350,000 substances that is updated quarterly. They also offer a range of educational services to the public and to health professionals. All of the centers provide for the medical profession, on a 24-hour basis, information concerning the prevention and treatment of accidents involving ingestion of poisonous and potentially poisonous substances. Toxic emergency calls should go to a local Poison Control Center, which can be located by consulting the inside front cover of your local telephone directory. The FDA Office of Consumer Affairs (87-062) has assumed responsibility for responding to requests for information formerly handled by the Poison Control Branch.

PRIMARY CARE INFORMATION

87-167   NATIONAL CLEARINGHOUSE FOR PRIMARY CARE INFORMATION (NCPCI)
Department of Health and Human Services
Health Resources and Services Administration
Bureau of Health Care Delivery and Assistance
8201 Greensboro Dr., Suite 600
McLean, VA 22102
(703) 821-8955

SERVICES: Established in 1983, the National Clearinghouse for Primary Care Information provides information services to support the planning, development, and delivery of ambulatory health care to urban and rural areas where there are shortages of medical personnel and services. The clearinghouse distributes publications focusing on ambulatory care, financial management, primary health care, and health services administration that will be of special interest to professionals working in primary care centers funded by the Bureau of Health Care Delivery and Assistance. Although NCPCI will respond to requests from the general public, its primary audience is health care practitioners and administrators.

PUBLICATIONS: Professional materials are available on federally funded community health centers, migrant health centers, childhood injury prevention programs, health education, financial management, sexually transmitted diseases, lead poisoning, administrative management, and clinical care. Bilingual medical phrase books and a publications list are also available.

PUBLIC HEALTH SERVICE PROGRAMS

87-168 PUBLIC HEALTH SERVICE (PHS)
Department of Health and Human Services
Hubert H. Humphrey Bldg., Rm. 725-H
200 Independence Ave., SW
Washington, DC 20201
(202) 245-6867 (Office of Communications)
(301) 443-1874 (Grants Management Branch)
(800) 342-AIDS (AIDS Information Hotline)

SERVICES: The Office of Communications provides information on PHS, its components, and its programs. General inquiries from the public and questions regarding the policies of the Office of the Assistant Secretary for Health, which oversees PHS, are answered or referred to one of the five agencies in the Public Health Service. The Grants Management Branch outlines policy issues affecting the award, administration, and monitoring of PHS discretionary grants and cooperative agreements. PHS provides information to the public on the prevention and spread of acquired immune deficiency syndrome (AIDS) through a toll-free telephone hotline. The Office of Communications also serves as the contact for the Healthy Mothers, Healthy Babies Coalition, an informal association of voluntary, professional, and governmental health agencies that seeks to improve maternal and child health through public education.

DATABASES: PHS is represented on an internal interagency committee that oversees the management and operation of the COMBINED HEALTH INFORMATION DATABASE (CHID). The committee comprises representatives of the following PHS programs, whose databases are components of CHID: the National Arthritis and Musculoskeletal and Skin Diseases Information Clearinghouse (87-013); the Center for Health Promotion and Ed-

ucation (87-115); the National Diabetes Information Clearinghouse (87-014); the National Digestive Diseases Information
Clearinghouse (87-015); the National Heart, Lung, and Blood
Institute (87-126); the ODPHP Health Information Center (87-
118); and the Veterans Administration Patient Health Education
Clearinghouse (87-188). The CHID file now includes subfiles
of eight important programs—Arthritis, Diabetes, Health Education, Digestive Diseases, High Blood Pressure, Health Information, AIDS School Health Education, and the Veterans Administration Patient Education Programs. The combined file is
accessible through BRS.

RADIATION PHYSICS

87-169 PHOTON AND CHARGED PARTICLE DATA CENTER
Department of Commerce
National Bureau of Standards
National Measurement Laboratory
Center for Radiation Research
Radiation Physics Bldg., Rm. C-311
Gaithersburg, MD 20899
(301) 975-5551

SERVICES: The center maintains a comprehensive database of information on the ionization, cross sections, and stopping power of electrons, positrons, protons, and other charged particles. Questions are answered concerning radiation penetration, radiation dosage, radiation effects, radiation shielding, radiology, and health physics. Use of the center's information resources is permitted for persons with a professional interest in the field.

RADIOBIOLOGY RESEARCH

87-170   **ARMED FORCES RADIOBIOLOGY RESEARCH INSTITUTE**
         (AFRRI)
         LIBRARY
         Department of Defense
         NMCNCR, Bldg. 42
         Bethesda, MD 20814
         (301) 295-1330

SERVICES: The institute's areas of interest include radiobiology, physiology, biochemistry, pathology, immunology, psychology, dosimetry, health physics, nuclear medicine, and medical physics.   The library provides reference services, makes interlibrary loans, and permits on-site use of its collection. Services are available to those with a need-to-know and whose user requirements can be processed on an "as time permits" basis.

HOLDINGS: The library's holdings consist of approximately 10,000 books, 250 periodical titles, and 100,000 government-sponsored technical reports in hard copy and microfiche.

PUBLICATIONS: *AFRRI Scientific Reports; AFRRI Technical Notes.*

RAPE

**87-171 NATIONAL INSTITUTE OF MENTAL HEALTH (NIMH)
ANTISOCIAL AND VIOLENT BEHAVIOR BRANCH**
Department of Health and Human Services
Alcohol, Drug Abuse, and Mental Health Administration
Parklawn Bldg., Rm. 18-105
5600 Fishers Lane
Rockville, MD 20857
(301) 443-3728

SERVICES: NIMH's Antisocial and Violent Behavior Branch responds to inquiries from researchers, the professional community, and the public; maintains a listing of rape prevention and treatment resources to help people locate services available in their community and to facilitate networking among those working in the field of sexual assault; and develops and disseminates materials.

PUBLICATIONS: Consumer materials are available on sexual assault, rape prevention, FBI crime statistics, and audiovisuals. Professional materials are available on research grants, funding sources, and medical training films (available on loan from the branch). A national directory of prevention and treatment resources is available, as are multimedia packages for use with adolescents and by community organizations (free five-day loan). Single copies of publications and a publications list are available free.

RESEARCH RISK PROTECTION

87-172   NATIONAL INSTITUTES OF HEALTH (NIH)
OFFICE FOR PROTECTION FROM RESEARCH RISKS
Department of Health and Human Services
Bldg. 31, Rm. 4B-09
9000 Rockville Pike
Bethesda, MD 20892
(301) 496-7005

SERVICES: NIH's Office for Protection from Research Risks administers DHHS policy for the protection of human subjects of biomedical and behavioral research and PHS policy for laboratory animal welfare through the development and implementation of regulations and a program of education and guidance. It answers inquiries, distributes copies of developing and final regulations, and conducts an educational program. Services are free to all users.

SCHIZOPHRENIA

87-173 SCHIZOPHRENIA RESEARCH BRANCH
Department of Health and Human Services
Alcohol, Drug Abuse, and Mental Health Administration
National Institute of Mental Health
Parklawn Bldg., Rm. 10C-16
5600 Fishers Lane
Rockville, MD 20857
(301) 443-4707

SERVICES: The Schizophrenia Research Branch, formerly the Center for Studies of Schizophrenia, serves as a focal point for coordinating NIMH activities in the psychological, social, and biological aspects of schizophrenias and related disorders, including their etiology, diagnosis, classification, treatment, epidemiology, and prevention. It collaborates with organizations within and outside NIMH to stimulate, develop, and support programs of research, service, demonstration, and training. Use of the branch's information services are limited to mental health professionals and researchers.

PUBLICATION: *Schizophrenia Bulletin* (quarterly journal).

SECOND SURGICAL OPINION

87-174 NATIONAL SECOND SURGICAL OPINION PROGRAM
Department of Health and Human Services
Health Care Financing Administration
Hubert H. Humphrey Bldg., Rm. 428H
200 Independence Ave., SW
Washington, DC 20201
(800) 638-6833
(800) 492-6603 (Maryland Only)

SERVICES: Established in 1978, the National Second Surgical Opinion Program is an information resource for people faced with the possibility of nonemergency surgery. It encourages the public to get a second opinion for nonemergency surgery. The Health Care Financing Administration is responsible for Medicare and Medicaid beneficiaries, and this program is especially directed to them. The program sponsors the government's toll-free telephone number to assist callers in locating a surgeon or other specialist. Files based on information requests are maintained.

PUBLICATION: A pamphlet is available which poses questions that a patient should ask and suggests how to find a specialist to get a second opinion. Write Surgery, Department HHS, Washington, DC 20201.

SLEEP

87-175 PROJECT SLEEP
Department of Health and Human Services
Alcohol, Drug Abuse, and Mental Health Administration
National Institute of Mental Health
Parklawn Bldg., Rm. 11-105
5600 Fishers Lane
Rockville, MD 20857
(301) 443-3948

SERVICES: A cooperative project funded by the Federal Government and the private sector, Project Sleep seeks to improve the diagnosis of sleep disorders, improve public knowledge of the problems, and identify research needs. Its principal areas of interest are the diagnosis and treatment of sleep disorders, insomnia, sleep apnea, hypnotic drugs, and sleep and aging. The project staff answers inquiries, provides reference services, conducts seminars and workshops, provides information on research in progress, distributes publications, and makes referrals to other source of information. Services are free and available to the public.

PUBLICATIONS: Pamphlets, posters, and other educational materials.

SMOKING AND HEALTH

87-176   **OFFICE ON SMOKING AND HEALTH**
          TECHNICAL INFORMATION CENTER
          Department of Health and Human Services
          Centers for Disease Control
          Center for Health Promotion and Education
          Parklawn Bldg., Rm. 1-16
          5600 Fishers Lane
          Rockville, MD 20857
          (301) 443-1690

SERVICES: The Office on Smoking and Health offers bibliographic and reference services to researchers through its Technical Information Center (TIC), which publishes and distributes a number of titles in the field of smoking and health and has the computer capability, through its Automated Search and Retrieval System, to generate comprehensive bibliographic printouts on topics of current interest on smoking and health. In addition to the bibliographic services offered, TIC recently initiated a Smoking Studies Section for the collection and analysis of numeric data sets, which contain significant tobacco use information. This section also designs and conducts national surveys on smoking behavior, attitudes, knowledge, and beliefs among adults and teenagers on a periodic basis, and works with other individuals and organizations that are interested in incorporating smoking behavior as part of their survey research activities. Visitors may use the collection weekdays from 8:30 a.m. to 5:00 p.m., EST. Advance arrangements for visits are suggested. Reference services are also provided by telephone. Copies of reference items can be provided in single copies only, and only in cases where materials cannot be obtained from other sources. Search Request Forms should be used to request free literature search service from the center. TIC also serves as the World Health Organization collaborating center for health information on smoking, tobacco, and tobacco use.

DATABASE: The online SMOKING AND HEALTH database contains approximately 50,000 bibliographic records dating mostly from the 1960s to the present, with selective material for the period from 1900 to 1950. The file includes citations and abstracts of the worldwide literature on all health aspects of smoking, tobacco, and tobacco use. Source materials indexed in the file include technical reports, scientific journals, monographs, books, book reviews, annual reports, and patents. Beginning in February 1987, the database became available to the public through DIALOG.

PUBLICATIONS: Consumer materials are available on smoking and teenagers, smoking and pregnancy, smoking cessation, and smoking and health. Professional materials are available on smoking, cancer, heart diseases, and lung diseases. *Smoking and Health Bulletin* (bimonthly); *Bibliography of Smoking and Health* (annual); *Health Consequences of Smoking* (annual report of the Surgeon General); and *State Legislation on Smoking and Health* (annual). Copies of the 1968 through 1985 editions of the annual *Bibliography* are available while supplies last; the 1986 edition is in preparation. A publications list also is available.

SOCIAL SECURITY BENEFITS

**87-177 SOCIAL SECURITY ADMINISTRATION
LIBRARY**
Department of Health and Human Services
6401 Security Blvd.
Baltimore, MD 21235
(301) 594-1650

SERVICES: The library's principal areas of interest are social insurance, health insurance, personnel and administrative management, hospital and medical economics, electronic data processing, social legislation, law, supervision and training, and operations research. Reference services and direct loans are restricted to Social Security Administration staff nationwide. Others may use the materials on-site if they are not available elsewhere. Materials are available to public and private institutions through interlibrary loan only. Limited copying service is provided.

**87-178 SOCIAL SECURITY ADMINISTRATION
OFFICE OF INFORMATION**
Department of Health and Human Services
6401 Security Blvd.
Baltimore, MD 21235
(301) 594-1988

SERVICES: Inquiries on Social Security programs can be directed to this office. At a local level, inquiries can be made to any Social Security office.

PUBLICATIONS: Consumer materials are available on Social Security benefits, Supplemental Security Income, and Medicare.

SURGICAL RESEARCH

87-179 **ARMY INSTITUTE OF SURGICAL RESEARCH**
Department of the Army
Office of the Surgeon General of the Army
Army Medical Research and Development Command
Bldg. 2653, SGRD-US
Fort Sam Houston, TX 78234
(512) 221-4559

SERVICES: The Army Institute of Surgical Research conducts clinical and laboratory studies and training programs in the treatment of seriously burned and injured patients, infection, renal failure, postburn endocrinology and immunology, metabolic changes, and effects of hyperalimentation. It provides technical answers, referral, and interlibrary loans to Department of Defense organizations, other governmental agencies, and medical and educational institutions, subject to facility and personnel limitations.

PUBLICATIONS: The institute's research reports are published annually and are available for a fee from the National Technical Information Service, Springfield, VA 22161.

TOXICOLOGY

87-180 HAZARDOUS SUBSTANCES DATA BANK (HSDB)
Oak Ridge National Laboratory
Information Research and Analysis Section
Biology Division
Bldg. 2001 (MS-50)
P.O. Box X
Oak Ridge, TN 37830
(615) 574-7587

SERVICES: The HAZARDOUS SUBSTANCES DATA BANK (HSDB), known as the TOXICOLOGY DATA BANK (TDB) prior to 1986, is sponsored by the Toxicology Information Program of the National Library of Medicine (NLM) (87-182). The Oak Ridge National Laboratory provides NLM with major input into HSDB in the laboratory's areas of interest, which are: toxicology research, including industrial, preventive, veterinary, and environmental toxicology and toxicology data extraction; biomedical research; ecological research; pathology research; pharmacology, drugs, and drug metabolism; environmental and occupational exposure hazards; environmental standards and criteria; epidemiology research analysis; food additives; industrial hygiene; personnel exposure hazards and monitoring; mammalian metabolism; pesticides; and carcinogens, mutagens, and teratogens. The laboratory staff answers inquiries, provides advisory and current-awareness services, evaluates data, and makes referrals to other sources of information. Services are available to the public.

The HAZARDOUS SUBSTANCES DATA BANK (HSDB) is a factual, nonbibliographic databank that focuses on the toxicology of potentially hazardous chemicals. It is enhanced with data from such related areas as emergency-handling procedures, environmental fate/exposure potential, detection methods, and regulatory requirements. Data are derived from a variety of books, monographs, and open scientific literature sources, as well as government documents and special reports. HSDB contains complete references for all data sources utilized. It is fully peer reviewed by the Scientific Review Panel (SRP), a committee of experts drawn from the major subject disciplines within the databank's scope. HSDB is an online interactive system, nationally and internationally available via the National Library of Medicine's TOXNET System (87-055). There are more than 4,100 records currently available in the HSDB public file.

87-181 NATIONAL CENTER FOR TOXICOLOGICAL RESEARCH (NCTR)
Department of Health and Human Services
Food and Drug Administration
Parklawn Bldg., Rm. 14-101
5600 Fishers Lane
Rockville, MD 20857
(301) 443-3155

SERVICES: NCTR, an interagency facility administered by the Food and Drug Administration, conducts research programs to study the biological effects of potentially toxic chemical substances found in man's environment. Its principal areas of interest are toxicological research and development studies to evaluate the effects of food additives, drugs, veterinary products, and environmental pollutants, including protocols for carcinogenicity, teratogenicity, mutagenicity, histopathology, and general clinical pathology; determination of adverse health effects resulting from long-term, low-level exposure to chemical toxicants; determination of basic biological processes for chemical toxicants in animal organisms; development of improved methodology and test protocols for evaluation of the safety of chemical toxicants; and development of data that will facilitate the extrapolation of toxicological data from laboratory animals to man. The center answers inquiries, provides information on

R&D in progress, evaluates data, and makes referrals to other sources of information.

87-182   **NATIONAL LIBRARY OF MEDICINE**
TOXICOLOGY INFORMATION PROGRAM (TIP)
Department of Health and Human Services
National Institutes of Health
Bldg. 38A, Rm. 3S-324
8600 Rockville Pike
Bethesda, MD 20894
(301) 496-1131

SERVICES: Established at the National Library of Medicine in 1967, the Toxicology Information Program (TIP) is responsible for the creation, development, building, maintenance, enhancement, and evaluation of a group of toxicologically oriented online databases that are part of NLM's MEDLARS (MEDICAL LITERATURE ANALYSIS AND RETRIEVAL SYSTEM) and TOXNET system (87-055). These databases contain either actual data or bibliographic citations received from governmental agencies, academic institutions, and professional associations, or obtained by contractual arrangement. In addition to making these databases publicly available, TIP's products and services include several publications and a query response service. The Toxicology Information Response Center (TIRC) (87-184), sponsored by TIP and located at the Oak Ridge National Laboratory, performs literature searches on request for a fee. TIRC also prepares specialized, annotated bibliographies on current topics in toxicology.

DATABASES: TIP's databases include TOXLINE and CHEMLINE, both available through MEDLARS (87-055). In addition, TIP has recently established the TOXNET system, which provides access to two more of its databases: the HAZARDOUS SUBSTANCES DATA BANK (HSDB) and the CHEMICAL CARCINOGENESIS RESEARCH INFORMATION SYSTEM (CCRIS). TIP provides financial support to the Oak Ridge National Laboratory to produce input for the HAZARDOUS SUBSTANCES DATA BANK (87-180).

Questions concerning any of the databases should be directed to TIP at the above address.

TOXLINE (TOXICOLOGY INFORMATION ONLINE) is a bibliographic database covering the pharmacological, biochemical, physiological, environmental, and toxicological effects of drugs and other chemicals. Almost all references in TOXLINE have abstracts and/or indexing terms and Chemical Abstracts Service (CAS) Registry Numbers. The TOXLINE database contains more than 1.7 million recent references, while older information is available in BACKFILES.

CHEMLINE (CHEMICAL DICTIONARY ONLINE) is an online chemical dictionary with more than 700,000 records. It contains chemical names, synonyms, CAS Registry Numbers, molecular formulas, NLM file locators, and limited ring information. By providing synonyms and CAS Registry Numbers, which can significantly increase retrieval, CHEMLINE assists the user in searching other MEDLARS databases. CHEMLINE can also be searched to locate classes of chemical substances.

TOXNET (TOXICOLOGY DATA NETWORK) is a computerized system of toxicologically oriented databanks operated by NLM in parallel with MEDLARS. This minicomputer-based system includes a variety of modules used by NLM and its contractors to build and review records. For outside users, TOXNET offers a sophisticated search and retrieval package that permits efficient access to valuable data, drawn from numerous sources, on potentially toxic or otherwise hazardous chemicals. Currently, TOXNET consists of two online databases: the HAZARDOUS SUBSTANCES DATA BANK and the CHEMICAL CARCINOGENESIS RESEARCH INFORMATION SYSTEM. The HAZARDOUS SUBSTANCES DATA BANK (HSDB), sponsored by the National Library of Medicine and maintained by the Oak Ridge National Laboratory, Information Research and Analysis Section, Biology Division (87-180), was known as the TOXICOLOGY DATA BANK (TDB) prior to 1986. HSDB is a factual, nonbibliographic data bank focusing on the toxicology of potentially hazardous chemicals. It is enhanced with data from such related areas as emergency-handling procedures, environmental fate, human exposure, detection methods, and regulatory requirements. Data are derived from a core set of standard texts and monographs, government documents, technical reports, and the primary journal literature. HSDB contains complete references for all data sources utilized. It is fully peer-reviewed by the Scientific Review Panel (SRP), a committee of experts drawn from the major subject disciplines within the databank's scope. HSDB is organized by chemical record, with more than 4,100 chemical substance records in the file. The CHEMICAL CARCINOGENESIS RESEARCH INFORMATION SYSTEM (CCRIS), developed and maintained by the National Cancer Institute, is a scientifically evaluated and fully referenced databank derived from both short- and long-term bioassays. Studies relate to carcinogens, tumor promotors, mutagens, cocarcinogens, metabolites, and inhibitors of carcinogens. Test results are reviewed by experts in carcinogenesis. Data are obtained from scanning primary journals, current-awareness tools, and a special core set of sources, including a wide range of NCI reports. CCRIS is organized by chemical record and now contains some 1,200 records.

87-183   NAVAL MEDICAL RESEARCH INSTITUTE (NMRI) TOXICOLOGY DETACHMENT
Department of the Navy
Naval Medical Research and Development Command
Bldg. 433, Area B
Wright-Patterson Air Force Base, OH 45433
(513) 255-6058

SERVICES: The Toxicology Detachment's areas of interest are the toxicology of chemicals of Navy interest; air pollution; hyperbaric toxicity; and the toxicity of propellants, oxidizers, hydraulic fluids, explosives, fossil-derived fuels, shale-derived fuels, and antifouling coatings. It will provide answers to inquiries or referral services.

PUBLICATIONS: The institute produces letter reports and publishes articles in the scientific literature.

**87-184   TOXICOLOGY INFORMATION RESPONSE CENTER
(TIRC)**
Oak Ridge National Laboratory
Information Research and Analysis Section
Biology Division
Bldg. 2001
P.O. Box X
Oak Ridge, TN 37831-6050
(615) 576-1743

SERVICES: TIRC is an international center for toxicology and related information, founded in 1971 by the National Library of Medicine's Toxicology Information Program (87-182). It functions within the Information Research and Analysis Section, a major scientific and technical unit of the Biology Division of the Oak Ridge National Laboratory. TIRC provides extensive toxicology information services to the scientific, administrative, and public communities on individual chemicals, chemical classes, and a wide variety of toxicology-related topics. It compiles comprehensive literature packages tailored to a user's specific request on a fee-for-service basis. Computer-associated charges, reproduction costs, and use fees for copyrighted materials are assessed, in addition to an hourly charge. Governmental agencies may consider interagency agreements. Response times vary from an immediate telephone answer to 8 to 12 days for computerized database searching to 3 to 4 weeks for in-depth literature searches. TIRC's multidisciplinary staff members provide search results in a variety of formats: specific published toxicology data, individualized literature searches, topical bibliographies, annotated and/or keyworded bibliographies, state-of-the-art overviews, custom searches of computerized data systems, and current-awareness service. Requests for information or searches may be submitted by letter or telephone.

PUBLICATIONS: Selected reports of topical concern are prepared and made available through the National Technical Information Service, Springfield, VA 22161. Publications sponsored by the Information Response to Chemical Concerns (IRCC)

Project are available through the Federation of American Societies for Experimental Biology, Bethesda, MD 20814. Publication lists and fact sheets are available from the center on request.

TROPICAL MEDICINE

87-185 GORGAS ARMY HOSPITAL
SAMUEL TAYLOR DARLING LIBRARY
Department of the Army
Health Services Command
Medical Department Activity, Panama
APO Miami, FL 34004

Located at: Ancon, Panama

SERVICES: The library's primary areas of interest are medicine and related sciences, with special emphasis on tropical medicine. The library answers queries, provides reference and literature-searching services, and permits on-site use of its organized information collection.

PUBLICATIONS: Bibliographies, including a *Fifty-Year Bibliography (1904-54),* covering medical activity in the Panama Canal Zone.

VETERANS MEDICAL CARE

87-186   VETERANS ADMINISTRATION (VA)
LIBRARY DIVISION
810 Vermont Ave., NW
Washington, DC 20420
(202) 233-3085

SERVICES: The division's principal areas of interest are medicine, dentistry, physical medicine and rehabilitation, nursing, dietetics, social service, rehabilitative research (prosthetics), veterans' benefits, alcohol and drug treatment, and allied health education. It serves the information needs of all headquarters components and supports and coordinates the Veterans Administration Library Network (VALNET). A total of 175 VA libraries make up the network: 166 VA Medical Centers, of which 6 have 2 divisions and 2 have outpatient facilities, and the Headquarters Library. Each library in the network has two principal responsibilities: to provide the clinical and administrative reference, bibliographic, and other information and audiovisual services required by the individual health care facilities of which they are a part, and to provide health information and recreational and educational materials for patients. In addition, all the libraries have a third responsibility, which falls most heavily on the libraries of the 136 VA Medical Centers that are affiliated with medical schools: to support the educational and research projects and programs of the Department of Medicine and Surgery by serving as comprehensive learning resource centers. The libraries answer queries, provide reference and interlibrary loan services, and permit on-site use of their collections. Except for literature-searching services, services to those outside the VA community are free and are provided as available resources permit.

87-187   VETERANS ADMINISTRATION (VA)
Office of Communications and Inquiries
810 Vermont Ave., NW
Washington, DC 20420
(202) 233-5081

SERVICES: The Veterans Administration was established in 1930 to provide a wide range of veterans' benefits in such areas as health care, education, housing, disability, pensions, and life insurance. Through its network of hospitals, clinics, and nursing homes, the VA provides a full range of medical care, long-term care, and patient support services. Veterans with service-related illnesses or injuries receive priority for VA medical services, and special consideration is also given to veterans who are in financial need, are over 65 years old, or are holders of the Congressional Medal of Honor. The VA is also involved in medical research and the training of health professionals. Training programs include graduate, undergraduate, and continuing education. Assistance for health manpower training institutions is also provided. VA benefits are restricted to U.S. military veterans.

PUBLICATIONS: Consumer materials are available on veterans' medical benefits and programs. Audiovisual medical training materials are available to professionals.

87-188   VETERANS ADMINISTRATION (VA)
PATIENT HEALTH EDUCATION CLEARINGHOUSE
Office of Academic Affairs (142E)
810 Vermont Ave., NW
Washington, DC 20420
(202) 233-3842

SERVICES: The VA Patient Health Education Clearinghouse, established in 1986, collects from VA medical centers descriptions of VA-designed Patient Health Education (PHE) programs. Each description, in addition to an abstract, contains a statement of program goals, methods/strategies, print/nonprint materials, and availability. The program descriptions are cataloged, indexed, and converted into machine-readable records for computer searching. Copies of the health education program materials described in the resultant database are available through interlibrary loan from the individual VA medical centers that prepared the requested programs.

DATABASE: The VA PATIENT HEALTH EDUCATION database is a new online component, as of March 1987, of the COMBINED HEALTH INFORMATION DATABASE (CHID) and can be accessed through BRS. It contains cataloged and indexed program descriptions of VA-designed PHE programs. The database presently contains 50 patient health education programs, with others scheduled to be added throughout the year.

Appendix
Databases Described in FHIR

ABLEDATA

An online database of the National Rehabilitation Information Center (NARIC) (87-024) that contains information about more than 4,000 commercially available rehabilitation products and aids useful to disabled persons, as well as a network of information brokers. Manufacturers of products for the disabled and those seeking product information are encouraged to utilize the ABLEDATA system.

AGRICOLA (AGRICULTURAL ON-LINE ACCESS)

The National Agricultural Library's (87-082) online bibliographic database, which provides access to the worldwide literature on agriculture. Its broad subject scope also highlights food and nutrition. In the United States, online access is available through BRS and DIALOG.

AIDS SCHOOL HEALTH EDUCATION

The Center for Health Promotion and Education (CHPE) (87-115) is developing this online database, which contains programs, curricula, guidelines, policies, regulations, and materials. It is part of the COMBINED HEALTH INFORMATION DATABASE (CHID), accessible online through BRS.

AIRLINE CABIN SAFETY

Data on in-flight and emergency evacuation injuries of passengers and crew members is contained in this computerized in-house database of the Civil Aeromedical Institute (CAMI), FAA (87-004). Inquiries should be sent to the institute.

AIR TRAFFIC CONTROL SPECIALIST

A computerized in-house database of the Civil Aeromedical Institute (CAMI), FAA (87-004), containing data of medical interest to the institute on air traffic control specialist selection, training, and tracking. Inquiries should be addressed to the institute.

ALCOHOL INFORMATION

An in-house bibliographic database established in 1972 and maintained by the National Clearinghouse for Alcohol Information (NCALI) (87-011). It includes abstracts of 50,000 items from scholarly journals, books, and statistical data. Access to the database is through NCALI.

ANTIBIOTICS, ANTITUMOR, AND ANTIVIRAL NATURAL PRODUCTS

A computerized in-house database of antibiotics, antitumor, and antiviral products that contains more than 10,500 compounds. The database is maintained by the Fermentation Program of the Frederick Cancer Research Facility, NCI (87-032). Comparison of unknown compounds with entries can be made using physical and descriptive characteristics. Service is available to scientific groups for a fee. Queries should be addressed to the facility in Frederick, Maryland.

ARTHRITIS INFORMATION

An online database, begun in 1979, that now includes records for more than 5,000 documents published since 1975; approximately 1,000 records are added each year. A thesaurus is used to index the entries. The file is part of the COMBINED HEALTH INFORMATION DATABASE (CHID), accessible to the public through BRS. The database is maintained and updated by the National Arthritis and Musculoskeletal and Skin Diseases Information Clearinghouse (87-013), operated for the National Institute of Arthritis and Musculoskeletal and Skin Diseases (87-016).

AUDIOVISUAL MATERIALS

An in-house computerized databank, maintained by the National Audiovisual Center (87-116), that contains information on audiovisual materials produced by the Federal Government that are available to the public.

AVLINE (AUDIOVISUALS ONLINE)

An online database of the National Library of Medicine (NLM) (87-055) that contains bibliographic citations of more than 14,000 audiovisual teaching packages (available on loan from NLM's Audiovisual Resources Section, 87-111) covering subject areas in the health sciences and cataloged by NLM since 1975. In some cases, review data such as rating, audience levels, instructional design, specialties, and abstracts are included. Procurement information on titles is provided. Access to the database is through MEDLARS.

BACKFILES (MEDLINE Backfiles)

The National Library of Medicine's (87-055) online database of five backfiles containing some 3.5 million older MEDLINE references (back to 1966). Access to the database is through MEDLARS.

BIOETHICSLINE

An online bibliographic database containing citations of documents that discuss ethical questions arising in health care or biomedical research. BIOETHICSLINE (87-055) is a comprehensive, cross-disciplinary collection of references to print and nonprint materials on bioethical topics. Included in the database are journal and newspaper articles, monographs, analytics, court decisions, and audiovisual materials. The database contains more than 19,000 citations from 1973 to date. Access is through MEDLARS.

BIOLOGICAL MATERIALS

A computerized in-house database maintained by the Cancer Treatment Program of the National Cancer Institute. The database contains raw and evaluated biological data on approximately 675,000 natural and synthetic materials. Queries should be sent to the Division of Cancer Treatment at the National Cancer Institute (87-031).

CANCER EDUCATION MATERIALS

A computerized in-house database of the Cancer Information Clearinghouse (87-028) that contains abstracts of and index entries to public and patient pre-1986 cancer information materials. Maintenance of the database was discontinued in 1986. Queries from health professionals and health educators should now be addressed to the Cancer Information Service (87-029).

CANCERLINE SYSTEM

CANCERLINE, a computerized system of the National Cancer Institute, consists of three separate databases: CANCERLIT, CANCERPROJ, and CLINPROT. CANCERLIT contains approximately 500,000 citations and abstracts covering the international cancer literature. CANCERPROJ contains descriptions of some 5,000 current cancer research projects around the world. CLINPROT contains summaries of approximately 5,000 clinical trials of new anticancer agents or treatment modalities. The total system is updated and maintained by the International Cancer Information Center (87-033) and is available for public access through NLM's MEDLARS (87-055). For more details on these databases, see descriptions of each in this Appendix or in 87-033 and 87-055.

CANCERLIT (CANCER LITERATURE)

An online bibliographic database, sponsored by the National Cancer Institute (87-033 and 87-055), that contains approximately 500,000 citations and abstracts of published international literature dealing with all aspects of cancer; it is updated monthly with some 5,000 abstracts. Approximately 80 percent of the literature is selected from an international collection of 3,000 biomedical and scientific journals. Nonserial literature (including books, reports, and meeting abstracts) contributes the remaining 20 percent. Informative abstracts averaging 200 words are included for most selected cancer-related documents. The database includes cancer literature from 1963 forward. Literature available for the period 1963 through 1976 is limited to references that had been selected for *Carcinogenesis Abstracts* and *Cancer Therapy Abstracts*. In 1977, the scope of the database was expanded to include all cancer-related literature, except most single case histories. In 1980, new records began including *MeSH* terms for uniform retrieval, and since January 1985, new records have been indexed with chemical names and CAS Registry/EC Numbers.

CANCERPROJ (CANCER RESEARCH PROJECTS)

The National Cancer Institute's online database of some 5,000 descriptions of current cancer research projects around the world (87-033 and 87-055). This file was reactivated in April 1985 and is expected to grow steadily, with quarterly updating, toward an eventual size of approximately 10,000 records. It contains descriptions of federally and privately supported grants and contracts. Twenty percent of the project descriptions are provided by scientists from outside the United States. The project summaries are usually divided into a statement of the research objective, a description of the experimental approach, and a statement of any progress made to date.

CANCER TREATMENT CLINICAL TRIALS

A computerized in-house database, maintained by the Cancer Treatment Program of the National Cancer Institute, that contains information on approximately 5,700 clinical trials worldwide. Queries should be sent to the Division of Cancer Treatment at the National Cancer Institute (87-031).

CATLINE (CATALOG ONLINE)

An online database of the National Library of Medicine (87-055) containing approximately 600,000 citations of books and serials cataloged by NLM. CATLINE provides medical libraries in the NLM network with immediate access to authoritative cataloging information, thus reducing the need for the libraries to do their own original cataloging. Libraries also find this database a useful source of information for ordering books and journals and for providing reference and interlibrary loan services. Access to the database is through MEDLARS.

CHEMICAL CARCINOGENESIS RESEARCH INFORMATION SYSTEM (CCRIS)

Developed and maintained by the National Cancer Institute (NCI), this online database is scientifically evaluated and fully referenced. It is derived from both short- and long-term bioassays. Studies relate to carcinogens, tumor promotors, mutagens, cocarcinogens, metabolites, and inhibitors of carcinogens. Test results are reviewed by experts in carcinogenesis. Data for CCRIS are obtained from scanning primary journals, current-awareness tools, and a special core set of sources, including a wide range of NCI reports. Organized by chemical record, the file now contains some 1,200 records. Access to CCRIS is through the TOXNET system of MEDLARS (87-055).

CHEMLINE (CHEMICAL DICTIONARY ONLINE)

The National Library of Medicine's (87-055) online chemical dictionary, which contains more than 700,000 records of chemical names, synonyms, Chemical Abstracts Service (CAS) Registry Numbers, molecular formulas, NLM file locators, and limited ring information. By providing synonyms and CAS Registry Numbers, which can significantly increase retrieval, CHEMLINE assists the user in searching other MEDLARS databases. CHEMLINE can also be searched to locate classes of chemical substances. Access to the database is through MEDLARS.

CHILD ABUSE AND NEGLECT INFORMATION

An online database maintained by the Clearinghouse on Child Abuse and Neglect Information (87-038). The database, begun in 1977, is updated semiannually and primarily covers materials produced between

1965 and the present. Sources indexed include approximately 8,600 published documents, 3,500 program descriptions, 100 descriptions of research projects, and 550 descriptions of audiovisual materials, as well as excerpts from current state and territorial child abuse and neglect laws, including the welfare, criminal, and juvenile court codes. The database is accessible to the public through DIALOG. A thesaurus is available for a fee.

CLINPROT (CLINICAL CANCER PROTOCOLS)

An online database, sponsored by the National Cancer Institute (NCI), that contains summaries of approximately 5,000 clinical trials of new anticancer agents or treatment modalities. Updated monthly, most of the protocols in CLINPROT (87-033 and 87-055) are provided by the Division of Cancer Treatment (87-031) of the National Cancer Institute, while the remaining protocols are provided by major U.S. cancer centers or sources outside the United States. Protocol summaries include the objective and an outline of the study, patient entry criteria, dosage schedules, dosage forms, and special study parameters. The name and telephone number of the study group chairman are provided. CLINPROT is designed primarily as a reference tool for clinical oncologists. Access to the database is through MEDLARS.

COMBINED HEALTH INFORMATION DATABASE (CHID)

An online Public Health Service (87-168) file that includes subfiles of eight information programs: Arthritis (87-013), Diabetes (87-014), Health Education (87-115), Digestive Diseases (87-015), High Blood Pressure (87-126), Health Information (87-118), AIDS School Health Education (87-115), and Veterans Administration Patient Education Programs (87-188). The combined database is available to the public through BRS.

DARPIS (DRUG ABUSE RESEARCH PROJECT INFORMATION SYSTEM)

Maintained by the National Institute on Drug Abuse (NIDA) (87-069), this in-house computerized database contains information about drug abuse research projects. It is accessible through NIDA's Office of Science.

DHHS PROGRAM EVALUATION

An in-house computerized database of the Policy Information Center of the Department of Health and Human Services (87-089) that provides access to program evaluations by subject and sponsoring agency, with custom printouts, including abstracts, available on request. Sources indexed by this database include 1,600 program evaluation reports. Continual updates add approximately 175 entries annually.

DIABETES INFORMATION

Patient education and professional materials can be found in this online database. It is a component of the COMBINED HEALTH INFORMATION DATABASE (CHID), accessible to the public through BRS. The database is maintained by the National Diabetes Information Clearinghouse (87-014), operated for the National Institute of Diabetes and Digestive and Kidney Diseases (NIDDK). Indexing is based on a thesaurus developed by the clearinghouse.

DIGESTIVE DISEASES PATIENT EDUCATION MATERIALS

The online bibliographic database of the National Digestive Diseases Information Clearinghouse (87-015), operated for the National Institute of Diabetes and Digestive and Kidney Diseases (NIDDK). The database, which contains information about the clearinghouse's patient education materials, is part of the COMBINED HEALTH INFORMATION DATABASE (CHID) and is accessible to the public through BRS.

DIRLINE (DIRECTORY OF INFORMATION RESOURCES ONLINE)

Available through the National Library of Medicine (87-055), this online directory of health information resources is based on information developed by the former National Referral Center of the Library of Congress and on approximately 1,000 descriptions of health-related organizations provided by the ODPHP Health Information Center (87-118). Information sources covered include clearinghouses, technical libraries, professional societies, foundations, and federal and state agencies. Access to the database is through MEDLARS. A thesaurus of health information terms is available from the clearinghouse for a small handling fee.

ENVIRONMENTAL TERATOLOGY INFORMATION

A computerized in-house database of more than 32,000 technically indexed, bibliographic references to the literature (journal articles, abstracts, symposia proceedings, books, dissertations, reports, editorials, reviews, methods papers) in the areas of testing and evaluation of chemical, biological, and physical agents, and dietary deficiencies for teratological effects in warm-blooded animals. Chemicals are associated with Chemical Abstracts Service (CAS) Registry Numbers for simplified information retrieval. The file is maintained by the Environmental Teratology Information Center (ETIC) (87-079), a component of the Oak Ridge National Laboratory. Access to the file is through ETIC.

FAMILY PLANNING INFORMATION

The 5,000 documents and audiovisuals indexed in this computerized in-house database include patient education materials and descriptions of patient education methods. The database is maintained by the Family Life Information Exchange (87-040).

GPO PUBLICATIONS REFERENCE FILE

An online bibliographic file, maintained by the U.S. Government Printing Office (GPO) (87-088), of documents published by GPO. Searchable fields include subject, title, author, and stock number. The file is used online at GPO and is accessible to the public through DIALOG and BRS.

HAZARDOUS SUBSTANCES DATA BANK (HSDB)

Prior to 1986, HSDB (87-180) was known as the TOXICOLOGY DATA BANK (TDB). It is sponsored by the Toxicology Information Program of the National Library of Medicine (87-182) and is maintained by the Oak Ridge National Laboratory, Information Research and Analysis Section, Biology Division. HSDB is a factual, nonbibliographic databank that focuses on the toxicology of potentially hazardous chemicals. It is enhanced with data from such related areas as emergency-handling procedures, environmental fate/exposure potential, detection methods, and regulatory requirements. Data are derived from a variety of books, monographs, and open scientific literature sources, as well as government documents and special reports. HSDB contains complete references for all data sources utilized. It is fully peer reviewed by the Scientific Review Panel (SRP), a committee of experts drawn from the major subject disciplines within the databank's scope. Organized by chemical record, HSDB now contains more than 4,100 chemical substance records. It is an online interactive system, nationally and internationally available through the National Library of Medicine's TOXNET system (87-055).

HEALTH EDUCATION

The Center for Health Promotion and Education (CHPE) (87-115) maintains an online database that contains information on health education programs in schools, rural and urban communities, medical care facilities and settings, and work environments. The database was established to support CHPE's technical assistance and capacity-building efforts in health promotion and education. It is part of the COMBINED HEALTH INFORMATION DATABASE (CHID) available online through BRS.

HEALTH FACILITIES

The Office of Health Facilities (OHF) (87-096) maintains a computerized in-house database that contains information on facilities obligated under the 20-year uncompensated care assurances program. The data captured for facility obligations begun after January 1959 include location, name, type of facility, date uncompensated service obligation expires, and Hill-Burton grant funds. Queries should be addressed to the Office of Health Facilities, a component of the Health Resources and Services Administration.

HEALTH INDEX

An in-house computerized database that is maintained by the Clearinghouse on Health Indexes (87-121) as an index to health statistics sources such as those found in journal articles, books, conference proceedings, government publications, unpublished materials, speeches, and descriptions of research in progress. The database is comprehensive since its origin in 1973 and includes coverage of core materials published earlier.

HEALTH INFORMATION

The ODPHP Information Center's (87-118) *Healthfinders,* a series of annotated resource lists on various health topics, are included, full text, in the HEALTH INFORMATION subfile of the COMBINED HEALTH INFORMATION DATABASE (CHID), available through BRS.

HEALTH PLANNING AND ADMIN (HEALTH PLANNING AND ADMINISTRATION)

This online database is produced cooperatively by the National Library of Medicine (NLM) (87-055) and the American Hospital Association. It contains more than 300,000 references to literature on health planning, organization, financing, management, manpower, and related subjects. The references are from journals indexed for MEDLINE and *Hospital Literature Index,* selected for their emphasis on health care matters. This database will eventually also contain references to nonserial items such as books and technical reports. Included in the database are selected citations from the HEALTH PLANNING INFORMATION database (87-108), which was maintained by the National Health Planning Information Center until November 14, 1986. Access to the database is through MEDLARS.

HEALTH PLANNING INFORMATION

An online file containing citations of approximately 27,000 documents. It was maintained by the National Health Planning Information Center (87-108) until November 14, 1986. Searches of the file can now be done through the NTIS database (87-087). In addition, a portion of the file has been integrated into the HEALTH PLANNING AND ADMIN file of the National Library of Medicine (87-055) and can be accessed through MEDLARS.

HEALTH RELATED ORGANIZATIONS

Maintained by the ODPHP Health Information Center (87-118), this online database contains approximately 1,000 descriptions of health information resources such as those maintained by information clearinghouses, technical libraries, professional societies, private foundations, and federal and state agencies. The database has been made available to the National Library of Medicine for inclusion in the library's online DIRLINE database (87-055), a directory of health information resources based on machine-readable descriptions provided by ODPHP and the former National Referral Center of the Library of Congress. Access to DIRLINE is through MEDLARS. A thesaurus of health information terms is available from the center for a small handling fee.

HIGH BLOOD PRESSURE INFORMATION

An online bibliographic database of references to more than 4,000 items relating to hypertension, dating from 1973. Since January 1985, the database has been a component of the COMBINED HEALTH INFORMATION DATABASE (CHID), accessible through BRS. The database is maintained by the High Blood Pressure Information Center (HBPIC) (87-124), a service of the National Heart, Lung, and Blood Institute. A thesaurus is used for indexing and accessing purposes. The HBPIC file contains descriptions of more than 600 documents, 20 percent of which are directed toward patient audiences and 80 percent toward professionals.

HISTLINE (HISTORY OF MEDICINE ONLINE)

An online database of the National Library of Medicine (NLM) (87-055) containing more than 70,000 citations of monographs, journal articles, symposia, congresses, and similar composite publications as published annually in the *Bibliography of the History of Medicine.* Its scope includes the history of medicine and related sciences, professions, individuals, institutions, drugs, and diseases of given chronological periods and geographical areas. Access to the database is through MEDLARS.

HUD USER

An in-house computerized information service of the Department of Housing and Urban Development (HUD) (87-009), designed to disseminate the results of research sponsored by HUD. Services include personalized literature searches of the database, document delivery, and special products such as topical bibliographies and announcements of important future research. Health-related topics include housing safety, housing for the elderly and handicapped, and lead-based paint. There is a handling fee for all documents ordered from HUD USER; please call for charges before ordering. Inquiries should be addressed to HUD USER, P.O. Box 280, Germantown, MD 20874-0284, or call (301) 251-5154.

HUMAN NUTRITION RESEARCH AND INFORMATION MANAGEMENT (HNRIM)

Announced in November 1986, this computerized interagency database, maintained by the National Institutes of Health (NIH) (87-148), provides information on 4,000 human nutrition research and research training activities supported in whole or in part by the Federal Government. Each participating agency (at present, the Department of Health and Human Services, Department of Agriculture, Veterans Administration, Agency for International Development, Department of Defense, and National Marine Fisheries Service of the Department of Commerce) assembles and submits its own data to NIH for merging into a central HNRIM database and updating on a quarterly basis. The database may be purchased from the National Technical Information Service, Springfield, VA 22161.

LOAN EARLY WARNING SYSTEM (LEWS)

The Office of Health Facilities (OHF) (87-096) maintains an in-house computerized database that uses key financial indicators to signal potential financial difficulties of facilities in receipt of DHHS direct and guaranteed loans and FHA-2442 insured loans. LEWS can also be used to examine the fiscal stability of loan applicants. Queries should be addressed to OHF.

MEDLARS (MEDICAL LITERATURE ANALYSIS AND RETRIEVAL SYSTEM)

This computerized system, based at the National Library of Medicine (87-055), is available through a nationwide network of more than 2,500 centers at universities, medical schools, hospitals, governmental agencies, and commercial organizations. MEDLARS is made up of multiple databases and contains some 8.0 million references to journal articles and books in the health sciences published after 1965. A user may search the store of references to produce a list of those pertinent to a specific question. Fact sheets and pocket guides describing the various databases are available. A MEDLARS management service desk at NLM is staffed to answer questions about the system.

MEDLINE (MEDLARS ONLINE)

An online bibliographic database of the National Library of Medicine (87-055) that contains approximately 800,000 references to biomedical journal articles published in the current and three preceding years. An English abstract, if published with the article, is frequently included. The articles are from 3,000 journals published in the United States and foreign countries. Coverage of previous periods (back to 1966) is provided by BACKFILES, searchable online, which total some 3.5 million references. MEDLINE can also be used to update a search periodically. The search formulation is stored in the computer; each month, when new references are added to the database, the search is processed automatically and the results are mailed to the user from NLM. Access to the database is through MEDLARS, BRS, and DIALOG.

NATIONAL ELECTRONIC INJURY SURVEILLANCE SYSTEM (NEISS)

A computerized system, maintained by the Consumer Product Safety Commission (87-058 and 87-063), that monitors a statistical sample of hospital emergency rooms for injuries associated with consumer products. The system is made up of 4 files: (1) coded reports on product-related injuries, (2) accident investigations conducted by staff members, (3) death certificates, and (4) consumer complaints.

NATIONAL LIBRARY OF MEDICINE/NATIONAL INSTITUTES OF HEALTH INFORMATION SERVICE

An online service of information on current clinical studies at the National Institutes of Health (87-052). Access to the database, an electronic bulletin board for health professionals, is through MINET (MEDICAL INFORMATION NETWORK), a service of the American Medical Association and GTE Telenet.

NIOSHTIC

An online database, maintained by the National Institute for Occupational Safety and Health, NIOSHTIC (87-156) indexes current and retrospective materials dating back to the 1800s, covering the field of occupational safety and health. Sources indexed by this database include journal articles, materials from the International Labor Organization's (ILO) Clearinghouse for Occupational Safety and Health, the International Occupational Safety and Health Information Center database, and references from *NIOSH Criteria Documents* and *Current Intelligence Bulletins*. The database is available through DIALOG.

NTIS BIBLIOGRAPHIC DATABASE

The NTIS Bibliographic Database is maintained by the National Technical Information Service (87-087), a component of the Department of Commerce. It is searchable online through the commercial vendors DIALOG, BRS, and SDC, or with NTIS assistance. The database consists of bibliographic citations or research summaries of the approximately 70,000 technical reports announced annually; it is updated biweekly and corresponds to the NTIS abstract journal *Government Reports Announcements and Index (GRA&I)*. Surveys indicate that the NTIS database is one of the most widely used databases in the world.

NUTRIENT DATA BANK

A system maintained by the Human Nutrition Information Service (HNIS) (87-084) that contains survey data on nutrient values in food and descriptions of the food. It creates for each an average value, which is incorporated into *Agriculture Handbook No. 8, Composition of Foods*. The system operates in batch mode. Although not searchable online, some summarized information from the databank can be purchased from the National Technical Information Service, Springfield, VA 22161.

PATIENT HEALTH EDUCATION

The Veterans Administration's (VA) PATIENT HEALTH EDUCATION database, maintained by the VA Patient Health Education Clearinghouse (87-188), became a new online component of the COMBINED HEALTH INFORMATION DATABASE (CHID) in March 1987 and can be accessed through BRS. It contains 50 cataloged and indexed descriptions of VA-designed patient health education programs, with others to be added throughout the year.

PDQ (PHYSICIAN DATA QUERY)

An online, interactive database that is sponsored by the National Cancer Institute (NCI) and is maintained by the International Cancer Information Center (87-033). It provides ready access to information on state-of-the-art and investigational cancer treatments and is designed to more effectively disseminate information on cancer treatment to the medical community. The PDQ database consists of three interlinked files, organized and internally arranged to facilitate interactive searching and retrieval by users. These files cover cancer information and treatment, a directory of physicians and organizations that provide cancer care, and active NCI-supported protocols from the CLINPROT file. To each of these approximately 700 research protocol descriptions, NCI has added a list of the institutions where the protocol is being used to treat patients and the name of an oncologist to contact at each institution for information about the protocol. The database is menu-driven, which makes it a "user-friendly" system for individuals who are inexperienced in using computers for online information searching. PDQ can be accessed through MEDLARS of the National Library of Medicine (87-055).

POPLINE (POPULATION INFORMATION ONLINE)

This online database is produced in cooperation with the Population Information Program of Johns Hopkins University; the Center for Population and Family Health of Columbia University; and the Population Index, Office of Population Research, Princeton University. It provides bibliographic citations to the worldwide literature on population and family planning and contains more than 100,000 citations and abstracts of a variety of materials, including journal and newspaper articles, monographs, technical reports, and unpublished works. Access to the database is through MEDLARS (87-055).

PROJECT SHARE

An in-house computerized file of current research and development activities, project descriptions, and accounts of the experiences of state and local governments in the planning and management of human services delivery. The file, which contains more than 12,000 records, is updated quarterly and covers the years since 1972. Abstracts are included for each record, and indexing is done using a taxonomy. Access to the database is through Project Share (87-092).

RAUS (RESEARCH ANALYSIS AND UTILIZATION SYSTEM)

An in-house database of the National Institute on Drug Abuse (NIDA) (87-069) that contains substance abuse research results. It is accessible through NIDA's Office of Science.

REGISTRY OF TOXIC EFFECTS OF CHEMICAL SUBSTANCES (RTECS)

RTECS is an online, interactive version of the National Institute for Occupational Safety and Health's (NIOSH) publication *Registry of Toxic Effects of Chemical Substances,* formerly called the *Toxic Substances List.* Maintained by NIOSH (87-157) and compiled annually, it contains basic acute and chronic toxicity data for more than 78,000 potentially toxic chemicals. Records include toxicity data, chemical identifiers, exposure standards, and status under various federal regulations and programs. The file can be searched by chemical identifiers, type of effect, or other criteria through MEDLARS (87-055).

REHABATA

An online database containing bibliographic information and abstracts of the National Rehabilitation Information Center's (NARIC) (87-024) entire collection of 300 periodical titles and more than 11,000 research reports, books, and audiovisuals, including materials produced from 1950 to the present. Direct access to the database is through BRS.

RTECS, *see* REGISTRY OF TOXIC EFFECTS OF CHEMICAL SUBSTANCES

SDILINE (SELECTIVE DISSEMINATION OF INFORMATION ONLINE)

An online bibliographic database of the National Library of Medicine (87-055) that contains all citations to the forthcoming printed edition of the monthly *Index Medicus.* Access to the database is through MEDLARS.

SERLINE (SERIALS ONLINE)

A computerized database of the National Library of Medicine (87-055) that contains bibliographic information on approximately 60,000 serial titles, including all journals that are on order or cataloged for the NLM collection. For many of these, SERLINE has locator information so the user can determine which U.S. medical libraries own a particular journal. SERLINE is used by librarians to obtain information needed to order journals and to refer interlibrary loan requests. Access to the database is through MEDLARS.

SMOKING AND HEALTH

An online file, maintained by the Office on Smoking and Health, Technical Information Center (87-176), that contains approximately 50,000 computerized bibliographic records dating mostly from the 1960s to the present, with selective material from 1900 to 1950. The file includes citations and abstracts of the worldwide literature on all health aspects of smoking, tobacco, and tobacco use. Source materials indexed in the file include technical reports, scientific journals, monographs, books, book reviews, annual reports, and patents. Beginning in February 1987, public access to the database became available through DIALOG.

SUDDEN INFANT DEATH SYNDROME

The Sudden Infant Death Syndrome Clearinghouse (87-045) maintains a computerized in-house database of bibliographic references to patient- and family-oriented print and audiovisual materials. Access is through the clearinghouse, a service of the Division of Maternal and Child Health.

SYNTHETIC CHEMICAL COMPOUND DATABASE

Maintained by the Cancer Treatment Program (87-031) of the National Cancer Institute, this computerized in-house database contains structural data on 400,000 synthetic compounds, of which, nomenclature information is available on approximately 265,000.

TERATOLOGY DATA EXTRACTION FILE

An in-house computerized database, maintained by the Environmental Teratology Information Center (ETIC) (87-079), a component of the Oak Ridge National Laboratory, that contains tabular abstracts of selected articles having specific details pertaining to experimental design, conditions, and observed effects. Access to the file is through ETIC.

TOXICOLOGY DATA BANK (TDB) *see* HAZARDOUS SUBSTANCES DATA BANK (HSDB)

TOXLINE (TOXICOLOGY INFORMATION ONLINE)

An online bibliographic database of the National Library of Medicine (87-055) that covers pharmacological, biochemical, physiological, environmental, and toxicological effects of drugs and other chemicals. It contains more than 1.7 million recent references, while older information is available in BACKFILES. Almost all of the references in TOXLINE have abstracts and/or indexing terms and Chemical Abstracts Service (CAS) Registry Numbers. Access to the database is through MEDLARS.

TOXNET (TOXICOLOGY DATA NETWORK)

A computerized system of toxicologically oriented databanks operated by NLM in parallel with MEDLARS (87-055). This minicomputer-based system includes a variety of modules used by NLM and its contractors to build and review records. For outside users, TOXNET offers a sophisticated search and retrieval package that permits efficient access to valuable data, drawn from numerous sources, on potentially toxic or otherwise hazardous chemicals. Currently TOXNET consists of two online databases: the HAZARDOUS SUBSTANCES DATA BANK (HSDB) and the CHEMICAL CARCINOGENESIS RESEARCH INFORMATION SYSTEM (CCRIS). The HAZARDOUS SUBSTANCES DATA BANK, sponsored by the National Library of Medicine and maintained by the Oak Ridge National Laboratory, Information Research and Analysis Section, Biology Division (87-180), was known as the TOXICOLOGY DATA BANK (TDB) prior to 1986. For more detailed information on HSDB and CCRIS, see descriptions of each in this appendix or in 87-055 and 87-180.

Agency / Organization Index

Subject / Title Index